ROUND 17 & ½

The Names Have Been Changed to Protect the Inefficient

Rich Siegel

DEDICATED TO SPIKE

I should be making this dedication to my wife and my family for allowing me the time to sit in my office and, without interruption, clack away at the keyboard until something of note, or at least the minimum words for a book, was produced.

This, I've heard, is the standard practice of many authors.

Then there's the obligatory acknowledgment of high school English teachers, advertising colleagues, and real world as well as digital friends who supported this effort with words of encouragement.

And if I had a literary agent, he or she too would be respectfully thanked, more so, if the check from the publishing company cleared the bank.

But the real gratitude belongs to my neighbor's dog, Spike.

A vicious, gnarling 75 pound Malinois Shepherd.

Mal being Latin for bad.

And *Nois* being French for noise.

Spike barks at anything that moves: cats, squirrels, moths, and crazy neighbors prowling the yard in their tighty whities with high pitch frequency iPhone apps that do little to deter barking.

In addition to being loud, he is foul-tempered.

One day, Spike bolted through the unlatched front door and locked his reptilian jaws around the neck of my unsuspecting and incredibly gentle golden retriever. If not for a good swift kick to Spike's head with the steely toe of my hiking boot, I would now be a grieving former pet owner.

In addition to his unprovoked assaults, this thoroughly untrained monster is fond of loudly doing his business at 4:47 A.M.

For the past year and a half, I have been awakened by Spike's incessant barking. And because I am now unable to go back to sleep, a useful skill I had in my youth, I decided to make the most of my involuntary early rising, and write.

Accordingly, this book is dedicated to you, Spike.

If not for you, I would have frittered away countless hours in deep REM sleep, dreaming of Scarlet Johansson and Megan Fox on a sex swing suspended from my high vaulted ceilings.

Now that the book is written, I would like to resume my normal sleeping pattern. Unfortunately, that's not on Spike's agenda.

I'm a dog lover and would never wish for his demise.

If however, Spike were to be hit by the #3 Culver City Green Line Bus near the corner of Braddock and Overland, and have all his ugly, serrated teeth knocked out, lose his larynx and his ability to bark, I might reconsider my militant stand on atheism.

Rich Siegel is also the author of *Tuesdays With Mantu, My Adventures with a Nigerian Con Artist.*

And blogs regularly at http://roundseventeen.blogspot.com

This is a work of fiction. Names, characters, businesses, places, events and incidents are either the products of the author's imagination or used in a fictitious manner. Any resemblance to actual persons, living or dead, or actual events is purely coincidental.

Printed in the United States of America

First Printing, 2015

ISBN 978-0-692-50758-2

Erupting Volcano Publications

www.eruptingvolcanopublications.com

Introduction

To enter the wonderful world of advertising, you must have a book ~ a portfolio of work demonstrating your ability to solve business problems with the creative use of pictures and words.

This is an exercise in faulty logic as most college graduates do not have the ideas or the skills to crack sophisticated marketing problems. Most still have a difficult time navigating the cooking instructions on a box of macaroni and cheese.

Nevertheless, a portfolio, or as it is commonly referred to, a book, is the price of entry.

Fittingly, a book is also the price of egress. At least in my case.

Allow me to explain.

If I am going to make the successful transition from advertising copywriter to ex-advertising copywriter, I'm going to need a source of income. I've heard there are millions of dollars to be made in the publishing of short stories. Millions.

And so I've dutifully captured the 25-plus years of brainstorming, ideating, conferencing, pitching, re-pitching, cross-country schlepping, late night pizza-eating, whoring, ass-kissing, bullet-dodging, back-of-the-plane sitting, and shameless soul-selling, and compiled them into a collection of fictionalized and overly-embellished short stories for your consumption and amusement.

And my retirement.

This is not exactly a swan song, because even after its publication I still hope to earn a living as a freelance copywriter, just as I have done for the past dozen years. I still command a healthy day rate. And it's hard to walk away from the noble, purpose-driven marketing work that keeps this Earth spinning on its axis.

I mean, if I don't make people pick up a phone and order a two-topping pizza for just $7.99, then who will?

There's also this thing called a time-space continuum. I won't bore you with the quantum physics, mostly because I can't, but I learned at a very early age how to tell time. And time is telling me, a 44-year-old freelance copywriter, to have plenty of nuts in storage for the cold wintry days of my incontinence ahead.

My greatest fear in life is to conclude this journey in a dirty nursing home. And knowing my luck, I'll end up sharing a room with an old codger named Maury, who suffers from dementia (not the funny kind). My imaginary roommate Maury will have the worst body odor. And still cannot dislodge a pesky gnat from his throat that has been stuck there since 1997.

Our filthy nursing home room will be tended to by Duron, a sticky-fingered Jamaican orderly who has a penchant for cashew nuts, spicy beef jerky or anything else, it seems, he can find in the care packages dropped off by my two loving daughters on their obligatory, bi-annual nursing home visits.

Duron, a man who can barely speak English, enjoys showing off "his" two Clio statuettes and three One Show Pencils that now sit on the coffee table of his Pacoima apartment.

I desperately want to avoid this awful scenario and so until this book lands me on Oprah's Book Review and the royalty checks roll in twice daily, I will continue to write Dealer Sales Event commercials, two-for-one eyeglass specials and banner ads for custom made catheters.

Because I need the money. And because I'll be damned if Duron is going to get his hands on my Western Region Silver Addy Award.

This book is not a tell-all, as the title might indicate.

I have a pet peeve with book titles. Too often, authors engage in obfuscation. Or bury the meaning of a book's title in subtext. I'm not a fan of either. It took me 176 pages before I realized J.D. Salinger's *Catcher in the Rye* was not about baseball. Or whiskey.

When I read, I do so in search of information or entertainment. If what I'm reading is too thick or convoluted I will, as I suspect many do, slap the covers together and put the book back on the shelf.

There are just too many good television shows digitally beckoning for my attention on the DVR.

And there's this thing called the Internet, where I can indulge my fascination for Beyoncé's involvement with the Illuminati, the Freemasons and the Rothschild Trilateral International Banking Cartel. Or fiddle away the hours watching videos of fanatical Muslim clerics talking about Israeli trained dolphin spies and pigeon assassins. Or troll websites that are rehashing *The Protocols of the Elders of Zion*, including the recipe for making matza with the fresh blood of gentile children.

"That's good matza, was this made with the Bergquist kid?"

Round Seventeen & 1/2 is a heavy-handed way to leverage the loyal readership of my blog, Round Seventeen, now in its seventh year.

As of this writing, the blog averages 10,000 views a month. Many of those hits are simply me going back to fix typos and malapropisms, nevertheless, it can be argued there is a built-in audience of suckers....er, loyal readers who, for some unknown reason, are willing to swim in my pool of vocational vitriol and neurotic self-effacement.

The blog has more than 1,300 entries and I could have very easily curated an assemblage of the best posts, hired an art director to design a fancy eye-catching cover and called it a day.

But I have no desire to rehash what has already been hashed. That would have put the vanity in vanity publishing.

This is all new material. Less ranting (a little less). More storytelling. Worthy, I hope, of earning some treasured real estate on your nightstand. Or, if I'm lucky, on the lid of your toilet.

The subtitle, *The Names Have Been Changed to Protect the Inefficient*, is self-explanatory. Or at least it should be.

I'm not at the point in my career, though I am looking forward to it, when I can name names and point an indignant finger at those who have earned that indignation. In other words, I'm not ready to set the proverbial bridge on fire. Though a healthy advance from Random House for my next book would get me there quickly.

Besides, and perhaps this is a troublesome sign of maturation, where's the fun in that? It's much more rewarding to indict the industry and those who have given the industry a bad name, with thinly veiled stories and inside-the-park references.

It should also be pointed out that the last thing I wanted to do was to put out another advertising memoir. The virtual bookshelves at Amazon are spilling over with dreary recollections of "that night we got stuck at the Memphis airport, the presentation got lost, Carol and Tom got drunk, and the next day the client was fuming mad, blah, blah, blah." I didn't want to waste my energy on that.

Finally, I'm somewhat familiar with this nation's laws regarding libel and slander. So, instead of putting the nest egg at risk, I've chosen to fictionalize my sleazy tales of low morals, sketchy ethics and no-talent poseurs engaged in endless peacocking. If any lawsuits were to arise, it should be noted, I'm carrying two mortgages, have two kids in college and wrongly invested all my money in the Microsoft Zune mp3 player.

Who am I kidding? This little inconsequential book will not put food on the table. And tomorrow I'll be right back at it. Writing corporate manifestos for automakers who believe their Blind Spot Detection System is more innovative than their competitor's Blind Spot Detection System. I'll be penning TV commercials for a mayonnaise company convinced their fatty sandwich dressing can change the world. And I'll be scheming up one of those Internet page takeovers that people just can't seem to get enough of.

The point is, I'll be working. Earning money. And saving money. Because I will not end up in a dirty nursing home nestled alongside the 605 Freeway.

Sorry, Duron.

If you want an advertising trophy, you're going to have to earn it the old fashioned way. You'll have to be sitting in the same room with the person who came up with the award-winning idea and find a way to finagle a slash.

CONTENTS

Life and Death in Room 112B

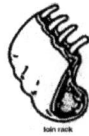

kein rack

Life and Death in Room 112B

The door burst open as if a bomb had exploded. The thundering force almost ripped the glass and wooden door from its industrial strength nickel-plated hinges. In the doorway, ready to pounce on anything that moved, stood portly, unknown copywriter Gerard Finnegan.

Unknown, though he was sure he had the chops to have his name spoken among the legends like Gossage, Hayden, and Fenske.

And portly, precisely because he was unknown, and had spent many a late night at the office where he took excessive comfort in soggy, thick-crusted pizza and slimy Pad Thai noodles.

His neck throbbed. His head turned on a swivel like a middle linebacker. He hardly looked like a sociopath, but one look at his bloodshot eyes and you could see all the wasted meetings with powerless middle managers. All the tedious and repetitive do-overs. All the accommodations to uninspired, ever-shifting strategic briefs that had come to define his career.

And now his face was splitting at the seams, like a twin-bearing woman in her 10th month of pregnancy.

Finnegan locked in on Aspirational Extrovert, a Data Analyst, 29, from Park Slope.

He could've picked Pragmatic Enthusiast, a Plumbing Supply Salesman, 34, from Bayside, who had earlier chimed, "I don't get it." And the equally insightful, "It's *too* creative."

2

But in a fleeting moment of rational thought, Finnegan had wisely made a mental note of the salesman's rather large forearms and well-calloused knuckles.

There was certainly enough reason to go after Youthful Influential, a Short Order Cook, 27, from Eastchester who had all but appointed himself Focus Group Table Captain. This hypercritical loudmouth had something to say about everything including the "overly wet tuna sandwiches."

A point, albeit the only one, Finnegan was willing to concede.

And of course there was Shirley, a crazy quilting lady from Garden City. Shirley didn't watch TV. She had retired her old Philco to the garage after the obscene 'wardrobe malfunction' of Super Bowl 38. No one, including Shirley, knew why she was even in the room.

But as the proprietor of A-1 Matrix Research explained, "By subjecting potential commercials to the deepest and most robust interrogation we offer our clients the best potential for market optimization and creative excellence." A dubious claim by a dubious expert who enjoyed having his publicity photo taken in front of a shelf full of equally dubious second-tier advertising awards.

Shirley, savoring the opportunity to be among people and voicing an opinion, claimed the commercial was "negative." Well, so was Apple's classic "1984" spot, Finnegan wanted to scream. But there were three good reasons not to pounce on Shirley. First off, she was a frail older woman.

Reasons #2 & #3: The extremely sharp quilting needles she held in each of her frail, old hands.

That's not to say that Aspirational Extrovert from Park Slope was picked by default. The anonymous 29-year old with an income of $75,000+ had it coming to him. He had annoying little personal tics that were exponentially magnified by the one-way mirror. When he wasn't mouth breathing, he was pooh-poohing the work.

"Why is that character a woman?"

"He should be wearing a blue shirt."

"That's not the way I would do it."

He did everything but suggest a monkey be in the commercial, a proposition heard in 43.7% of all focus groups.

His frame-by-frame criticism of the well-polished animatic could have, and should have, been immediately dismissed. But Aspirational Extrovert originally hailed from Streatham Hill, 12 km south of London. And clients are all too easily seduced by the intellectual lilt of the Queen's English, particularly when delivered by one of her native subjects.

It should also be noted that focus groups are attended by junior marketing executives. Senior marketing professionals do not waste their time at focus groups. They know from experience that there is more to be gained by staying home and watching an episode of "Wheel of Fortune."

"He's right," said the client, a perky Ad Manager, who four months earlier was busy organizing Spring Fling '14 for the Alpha Phi girls of Penn State. "We should totally rewrite the ending of the commercial."

Oh sure, let's rewrite the ending, thought Finnegan. After all, it's only 30 seconds. It only takes a few minutes to rewrite the end of a 30 second commercial. Conveniently neglecting the weeks, months and countless Xanax pills it takes to steward the new rewrites through the corporate maze of Gordian bullshit.

Fueled by adrenaline, Finnegan launched his portly body onto the conference room table. Bowls of M&M's, half-empty bottles of water and legal pads chockfull of homegrown marketing sagacity were unceremoniously tossed to the floor.

And the mood boards!!!

Those enlightening mood boards, with the preciously prepared pictures of men with sweaters tied around their necks and the coiffed women with lap dogs, that so succinctly redefined luxury for those who don't know what rich people look like, were all damaged beyond repair.

In a split second, Finnegan had slid the length of the table and throttled the unsuspecting Brit. With his newly gained weight he had no trouble wrestling the know-it-all to the ground. The first crushing blow was delivered before any of the $75-a-night-advertising experts in the room could jump out of their flimsy plastic chairs.

That stunning punch was followed by a flurry of others. Some hitting their mark. Others, wildly inaccurate. None of it mattered to Finnegan, who had unleashed not just one night's frustration on the unsuspecting Aspirational Extrovert, but an entire career's worth.

For the dog food campaign that got killed in 2003: a winding uppercut.

For the beer spot that failed to air during the Oscars: a short left jab.

For the ill-fated computer campaign that never got out of the agency: a glancing right cross.

The others tried in vain to pry Finnegan off the bloodied expatriate, but the writer seemed blessed with the power of a hundred men. If the bludgeoning had gone on five seconds longer, the coroner would have been summoned.

But fate, and a quick thinking Motivated Influencer, a Dental Hygienist from Yonkers, stepped in.

Life and Death in Room 112B

The 32-year-old Female, $45,000-$70,000, grabbed an award off the shelf of dubious awards and clocked the crazed copywriter on the head with the heavy metal base.

Finnegan fell to the ground. Fittingly cold-cocked by a Silver Clio that had been snagged from the Lincoln Center stage in the chaotic free-for-all of 1991.

Months later, significant sums of money, compliments of the Omnicom shareholders and Omnicom office holders who wanted to avoid bad publicity, changed hands. A deft lawyer successfully expanded the boundaries of temporary insanity and managed to convince a soft Upper West Side jury that under the enormous pressure of the day, and the pent up disgruntlement of years in the advertising industry, Gerard Finnegan simply cracked.

He left the ad business for good and opened a bed and breakfast alongside serene Racquet Lake in Upstate New York.

Had it not been for a fast-moving focus group attendee and a stolen advertising award, Finnegan would have been sitting on death row. He lived to win awards. And in the end, it was an award he didn't win that saved his life.

Nevertheless, he achieved what he had always hoped to achieve. He took a stand for artistic purity (if such a phrase can be used in conjunction with advertising). He earned the respect of his peers. And in doing so, joined the elite rank of copywriters who had made a name for themselves in the industry.

To this day, in moments preceding focus groups throughout this great land, nervous account executives can be heard whispering to demoralized writers, art directors, designers, "I know you hate these things and I know you don't want to be here, but whatever you do, please, please, don't pull a Finnegan."

Fill Up the Cup

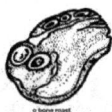

Fill Up the Cup

"There may be a problem with your sperm."

This was not the diagnosis Greenberg wanted to hear. He and Mrs. Greenberg had been trying to make a baby for the past two and a half years, since 1995. There were messy ovulation kits. Calendars. Vaginal thermometers. The tiny bathroom in their 3rd floor condominium could barely contain all the over-the-counter fertility paraphernalia.

And yet, for all their efforts, including the obligatory early morning *schtupp*, they had nothing to show for it. It was all a swing and a miss.

Mrs. Greenberg checked out fine. Her fallopian tubes were fallopianing. Her eggs were good, fertile eggs. And her plumbing system got the Good Housekeeping Seal of Approval.

Her lady doctor, who had called for the couple to come in for a joint consultation, pointed the finger at Larry Greenberg. More accurately she pointed the finger towards the region below his belt.

His first trip to a gynecologist went exactly as he thought it might.

If two and a half years of fruitless fornicating didn't make Greenberg self conscious about his virility, the accusatory sneer of his wife's (clearly) lesbian doctor surely did. She handed him a business card and instructed him to set up an appointment right away.

"Let's see what's going on down there."

Again she pointed to the area below his belt.

"Or, what's *not* going on down there."

Fill Up the Cup

Greenberg knew of the sperm banks discreetly located throughout the Westside of Los Angeles, but he had never been to one. When he first moved to California and took a room as a boarder at a UCLA fraternity house, he met some of the brothers who made a living at the local "whack shack."

They never studied. They never worked. They drank beer and smoked pot. And had plenty of money to fuel their pastime. All they had to do was walk down Gayley Ave., past the Chabad House, engage in some hand-to-gland combat and collect a check. They invited Greenberg to accompany them on one of their masturbatory sojourns, but he preferred to earn his money the old fashioned way – slaving as a dishwasher at the local Straw Hat Pizza.

Now, 15 years later, against all odds, he found himself in the lobby of the Beverly Hills Medical Services Laboratory. As he filled out the bundle of paperwork attached to the clipboard, his mind wandered.

The rational side of his brain knew that behind the locked doors he would not find a harem of short-skirted, leggy nurses ready to assist him with the precious extraction.

On the other hand, he was in Beverly Hills, a city known to indulge its residents, and suspected the lab had gone to extraordinary lengths to provide a comfortable, even posh, environment that would yield the maximum payload.

He envisioned plush, microfiber couches in a secure dimly lit room. A room endowed with the world's widest selection of pornographic stimuli. He even pictured a sleek, Japanese-designed custom electronic sleeve that would offer personalized, hands-free collection. The Tugatron 7000™.

All very conceivable for a sperm collection center located in one of the world's richest zip codes.

Fill Up the Cup

But Greenberg was wrong on all counts. Nurse Ratchet ~ he decided that was her name the second he saw her ~ came to the reception area and called out his name.

"Laaaaary. Laaaarrrry Greenberg."

She led him back behind a wall of clear acrylic that had the appearance and thickness of bulletproof glass. They zigzagged down a hallway lined with paintings, the kind of paintings you would only find in a medical laboratory hallway. The nurse opened the door to what looked to be a regular bathroom, an oversized regular bathroom with no special accommodations, with the exception of a tubular stainless steel handrail built to comply with the state's code for the handicapped.

"Wash and dry your hands thoroughly. Then, get it all in the cup."

"Wait, this must be a mistake," he thought.

"And no lubricant. None," she said before shutting the door behind her.

The room was exceedingly bright. The fluorescent light ricocheted off the cinder block walls. Dimensionally, it was not that far off from the standard two-person jail cell one might find at Folsom or San Quentin. There was nothing but a sink, a toilet, an all-aluminum table chair and a long narrow table that spanned the length of the tiny room.

Atop the table, there were three magazines.

They didn't put a lot of thought into the design of this room. Nor did they seem to consider its rather unique function. But at least they had the foresight to provide something in the way of visual stimulation.

Suddenly there was the roar of a toilet flush from the bathroom on the other side of the cinder blocks.

Fill Up the Cup

Greenberg looked at the three magazine covers spaced evenly across the long table.

The Economist

U.S. News & World Report

Harvard Business Review

One part of Larry Greenberg wanted to scream. The other, more sensible part of Larry knew that screaming would draw unwarranted attention and in effect say, "I can't make babies. Something is going on with my little men. So now I'm in a refurbished janitor's closet where they want me to dry hump myself into a little plastic cup!"

He didn't want to do that.

He locked the door. And then he threw the deadbolt into place. The last thing he needed was some overly inquisitive lab technician with a corridor key to accidentally walk in on him while he was flying solo.

He yanked about a dozen and a half paper towels from the dispenser above the sink, crumpled them up, wet them down, and stuffed them in the crevice between the bottom of the door and the floor stop. His mind raced with ugly possibilities. Somebody could be walking in the hallway, drop their car keys or a quarter, bend over to pick it up, peer through the crack under the door and spot Greenberg *solus in flagrante delecto.*

Not only could that happen, the way the morning was transpiring, Greenberg fully expected it to happen.

Acting out of extreme precaution, he pushed the featherweight aluminum chair against the back of the door. Greenberg would often tell people, "If he was in for a dime he was in for a dollar." And on

Fill Up the Cup

the issue of self-pleasuring privacy in a public setting, he was in for a buck seventy-five.

Before the mission began he took one last meticulous look at the cinder block wall. He slowly and carefully scanned the wall with the palm of his hand, delicately searching for any pinholes, where a hidden camera with a full battery and ample memory could be placed.

What if, again his mind raced, the Beverly Hills Medical Lab was an elaborate front? Maybe they were secretly selling footage of their patients masturbating? Could be an entire underground operation. Perhaps supplying the filthy tapes to fetishists in Cambodia? Or Laos?

Laos always seemed to Greenberg to be a place where old men, tired of the jungle, the red sticky mud, the constant monsoonal rain, and the day in/day out consumption of boiled monkey liver and rice, would entertain the notion of watching affluent and unsuspecting Americans jerking off behind closed doors.

Satisfied that the room was clean, it was time to get down to business.

Greenberg picked up the *U.S. News & World Report*. It was the magazine with the least written and the most photographic material. He threw it on the floor in front of him, undid the buckle of his pants and squatted on the cold aluminum chair.

In a feat of flexibility he did not know he had, Greenberg spread his legs wide, so that he could keep one foot solidly on the wall and the other wedged into the doorway, in case the lock, the deadbolt and the forest of wet crumpled paper towels did not suffice.

He fiddled through the pages hoping to find a picture of Madonna or Princess Diana, or some up-and-coming actress of the time, but could only find a spread on Queen Elizabeth. And an in-depth interview with Hillary Clinton.

12

Fill Up the Cup

Her Royal Highness was sporting a pink dress that bared the bottom half of her 70-year-old gams. The First Lady was wearing one of her signature pantsuits. Out of respect for the crown, Greenberg went with the younger lass from Arkansas.

A full 30 minutes later, the tug of war was over. Later, he joked he spent more 'sexy time' with Hilary Clinton than he had ever done with his own wife.

He gingerly screwed the cap on the plastic cup and placed it in the pass-thru vault, per the instructions of Nurse Ratchet. He double-checked the label on the cup. If some medical assistant were to make a mistake, he'd have to repeat the most humiliating, most joyless experience he'd ever had with his penis.

As he exited the clinic he drew his baseball cap tight across his brow in the hope no one would recognize him. The last thing he wanted was to run into a friend or a colleague and engage in some street side chitchat, particularly when he was sporting that telltale face that screams, "I just masturbated into a plastic cup."

From Beverly Hills, Greenberg drove a short 15 minutes to his office on Wilshire Blvd. He worked at one of the few remaining ad agencies that had not migrated west of Lincoln Blvd. They were an older, established shop with longstanding client relationships, relationships that had stood the test of time. And because they didn't suffer the wild fluctuations of revenue experienced by other agencies, they rarely had to engage in cutbacks or staff layoffs.

Greenberg grabbed some coffee and settled in behind his desk, hoping the rest of his day would be more routine.

"You're not going to believe this," said Sean Smithwick, Greenberg's management counterpart on the big Nestle account.

"What?" Greenberg shot back.

"They fired Anderson when they found out he was getting kickbacks from the printer. And they put in a new Chief Marketing Officer."

"Who?" said Greenberg.

"Get this. Coughlin."

"Who's Coughlin?"

"You know Coughlin, the girl that used to book all of Anderson's travel, do his timesheets and fill out his expense reports. Coughlin, his Executive Assistant."

"You gotta be kidding me. She's a CMO?"

"Who isn't a CMO these days?" said Smithwick. Adding, "Better strap in, buddy. Gonna get hairy here for the next few months."

Greenberg folded his arms over his desk and laid his head down for a much-needed rest.

A week later he and his wife were back in the offices of her gynecologist. The lady doctor mulled over the lab report. She did a line item check on every aspect of his manhood. And, as if to add to his agony, let him stew in silence as she carefully took notes and withheld his results. A second before he was about to explode...she cleared her throat.

"It seems the problem is not with you, Larry. Your boys are swimmers."

He breathed a sigh of relief. Not too heavy, because he didn't want his wife to notice. But inside, he was thrilled. If he could have high-fived his penis, he would have done so.

"In fact, and I'm wondering if there's some kind of mistake here. Your sperm count is unusually high."

Another high-five.

"Motility is..."

"Motility?" asked Larry.

"That's the sperm's ability to move. And yours is, again, unusually high, indicating raised levels of testosterone."

Larry could not help grinning. Particularly as all these results seemed to annoy the lady doctor to no end.

"In fact, many of your sperm cells have extra long tails, which we don't see that often."

"Long tails are good?" asked a very inquisitive Larry.

"For impregnation purposes, long tails are excellent. Frankly, these tests results are not at all what I expected."

If his wife had not been in the room, Larry would have taken little Lawrence out of his pants, laid it on the desk and not put it away until the doctor personally apologized. But his cell phone rang and there was an emergency back at the office that required his immediate attention.

"Before you go back to the office, I need you to stop by the Pico Robertson Lab for another sample," said the doctor.

"Another sample? I thought you just said my boys weren't the problem?"

"They're not. Which means we have to step up to a modified in vitro procedure. And we'll need to prepare your sperm for an injection."
"But I have to get back to work."

"You have some more important work to do first. Pico Robertson Lab. It's near Doheny."

Larry stopped at a newsstand. He wasn't going to have a repeat of his previous unpleasant experience with the *U.S. News & World Report*. He was going in prepared for the worst. Overcompensating, Larry reached to the top of the rack and grabbed a copy of the filthiest hardcore magazine he could find, *Slutty Sluts Get Their Slut On*. On the cover, a handcuffed woman in red leather chaps was being force-fed a foot-long Polish sausage.

He wouldn't need it.

The lab at Pico Robertson, in the heart of Little Jerusalem, was 180 degrees from the sterile surroundings in Beverly Hills. The nurse led him back to a room that looked unlike anything he had ever seen.

The walls were covered from floor to ceiling in black velour. The ceiling was covered with black velour. And the room was glowing with a purplish light from a small lava lamp tucked in the corner.

As he adjusted himself to the surreal, almost womb-like environment the nurse unveiled a credenza featuring a TV monitor, a VCR deck, and no less than 200 VHS tapes of the latest and greatest in porn offerings. The tapes had thoughtfully been arranged in alphabetical order and the selection covered everything from naughty threesomes to milfy MILFs.

The nurse smiled at Larry and left him to the business at hand.

He could hardly believe his good luck. He felt like a kid in a candy store. There was so much to choose from he didn't know where to start. Then he reminded himself that porn was porn. So he went for the first title that struck his funny bone, *Balling for Dollars*.

It had some vague connection to bowling and was a clear indication the pornmakers in the San Fernando Valley were running out of ideas. Nevertheless, there were a few steamy scenes of women in bowling shirts briefly getting frisky with the pin-chasers working the machinery behind the alleys.

Upon completion of his duties Greenberg gave serious thought to taking a nap, waking up 20 minutes later and going at it for another round. He had his eye on another movie, *In and Out of Africa*. Why let all this black velour go to waste, he figured. Why not shock the doctor and fill the cup all the way to the top?

His phone rang. It was Smithwick.

"Where the hell are you? And what's that moaning?"

"I'll be there in 10 minutes."

Greenberg drove back to the office along Pico Blvd. where the sidewalks were teeming with large Orthodox Jewish families. Many of the moms were pushing strollers. Behind the strollers there were often gaggles of little girls in long dresses and skinny little boys sporting thick black wool coats and exposed tzitzits. This backward lot of 19th-Century holdouts seemed to be fruitful. They were certainly multiplying. Why, he wondered, were he and Mrs. Greenberg unable to make another Greenberg?

"Coughlin's on a rampage." said Smithwick. "She wants to know why our Coffee-Mate flavored creamers are not selling in the Midwest and the Northwest territories."

"They're not selling because they taste like shit. And they're expensive. And people are buying their coffee in coffee shops," Greenberg offered.

"You want to tell her that? Or you want to run home and pack a bag? Because we're on a plane tonight for a whirlwind tour of the regional offices," said Smithwick.

"Tonight?"

"Hello, Boise."

The next day, Greenberg found himself, with Smithwick and Karen Coughlin, at the Super KMart on the outskirts of Boise. The store was the size of three football stadiums. And sold everything under the sun. Greenberg never understood the novelty of buying your breakfast cereal where you also buy your shotgun ammo.

As the store manager was showing the trio the exclusive end cap aisle display for Nestle Coffee Mate Flavored Creamers, he got a call from his wife. There was a mix up at the Pico Robertson lab and the label on his cup of sperm fell off.

Mrs. Greenberg did not go into too many details. She said what was done, was done. They had to deal with the present. And the present was pressing, as her ovulation kit indicated, time was of the essence.

"The doctor put me in touch with a company that does overnight delivery of medical supplies and equipment." said Mrs. Greenberg. Adding, "They have special freezing techniques."

"What?" said Larry.

"I want you to buy a small piece of Tupperware, go back to the hotel, fill the Tupperware, seal it and rush it over to their facility near the airport."

"You're not serious, are you?" asked Larry.

"Do I sound *not* serious?"

Larry wrote down the instructions and was careful to get every detail. He got off the phone and waited for the Super K Mart retail manager to finish his spiel.

18

"If we add the shelf talkers, I'd recommend the K9000 Series, we think we can increase floor traffic and impulse sales by 27%. You could have your own island of caffeination domination."

"That's excellent," said Ms. Coughlin.

"Of course it all depends on having the right messaging," added the manager.

"Listen, this is all very encouraging and fascinating too, but I have an emergency and have to get back to the Comfort Suites," said Larry.

Karen was not happy. "This is important stuff, Larry."

"It is. And I'd like nothing more than to find new ways of moving the Happy Hazelnut, but like I said it's an emergency."

"The Happy Hazelnut, the Vivacious Vanilla and the Mucho Mocha are kind of emergencies, too."

"I understand that, Karen."

"I'm not sure you do, Larry," she pressed. "What is so urgent that you need to rush back to the hotel?"

"It's a motel not a hotel because your efficiency expert keeps nickel and diming us, so let's be clear on that. And if you really must know, I need to go back to the motel to masturbate into a little plastic cup."

Larry realized immediately that he was not using his 'inside voice' and many Super KMart shoppers, who had come for the discounted shoes, bulk mayonnaise and two-for-one specials on tube socks, were going home with quite a story to share with friends and family.

An hour later, Larry found himself in the rental car rushing to the airport with his clearly labeled 'sample' of little Larrys tucked beneath his T-shirt which, according to his wife, would maintain the proper

Fill Up the Cup

temperature until it was flash frozen and put on a plane back to Los Angeles.

As he navigated through a fortunate string of green lights his imagination got the worst of him. What if he were to be T-boned by an oncoming car? The first responders would arrive on the scene to find his body covered in glass shards, caked blood and fresh semen. That wouldn't play well in the papers. And his snarky advertising friends would have a field day.

A Hit Jerk & Run, the headlines would shout.

He eased up on the gas pedal, tightened his seat belt and made a much more attentive check of all his mirrors.

Larry's boys successfully made the trip from Boise to Los Angeles. They did not, however, complete the journey and finish the last 1/,1,000,000th of a mile to fertilize Mrs. Greenberg's egg.

The next few months were not kind to Larry Greenberg.

He was doing his best to stave off an account review. That meant endless visits to supermarkets and big box grocery warehouses. Not to mention after-hours research at focus groups, where casual coffee drinkers would drone on about their choice of coffee creamers. A low interest category if there ever was one. Larry was convinced he had discovered the 8th Gate of Hell.

The 9th was not that far behind.

His tour of Southern California's Whack Shacks grew wider and wider. If there was anything more humiliating than walking into a building, signing some paperwork and then being led off to a room – in most cases by a woman – to milk yourself, he couldn't imagine what it would be.

Fill Up the Cup

On a cold, rainy Sunday morning, Larry found himself snuggled under the covers, looking forward to a hearty breakfast of salty lox, onion bagels and fresh whitefish salad. This would be followed by a lazy day on the couch watching football. Napping. Noshing. And watching more football.

Mrs. Greenberg had just gone to the bathroom. With his head buried under the pillow, Larry could make out the sounds of her unwrapping an ovulation detection kit. He detested that sound. Minutes later, she emerged from the bathroom. And heeding the unmistakable advice of her urine, told him it was once again time to do the one-handed gland dance.

He threw on a pair of sweat pants, went to the computer and found the only clinic that opened their doors on Sunday for *jizzness*. He grumbled to himself and started to brew a pot of coffee. But Mrs. Greenberg intervened.

"There's no time for that."

She nuked what was left in the carafe and shoved him out the door.

As sperm collection centers went, this one, on the north side of Santa Monica, was unusually small. It was almost impossible to find the office, with not much in the way of signage. When Larry walked in it was quiet. A tall blond woman with long, fire-red fingernails sat behind the desk. Suddenly he was not sure that sweatpants had been the right choice of attire.

He smiled at her, she smiled back and handed him a clipboard with a one-page form to fill out. Then she stood up from the counter and led him down the hallway.

"Follow me."
She was a full four inches taller than Greenberg. He couldn't keep his eyes off her legs. Or the black heels she was wearing. They weren't tall enough to be classified as cheap or trashy, but they were too tall for a

Fill Up the Cup

Sunday morning, particularly a Sunday when he hadn't shaved and was wearing a moth-eaten T-shirt.

She led him to a small room and handed him a small plastic cup. He made sure his hand brushed up against hers and wisely made the decision *not* to crack a joke...

"I might need a bigger specimen cup."

She pointed out the TV and told him to take as much time as he needed. She closed the door and in a ritual that had become familiar to Greenberg, he double bolted the locks and made sure no one was getting in unannounced.

Greenberg made himself as comfortable as possible. And suddenly the TV screen was flickering. There were no tapes. No awkward choices to make. The porn was simply piped in.

Seven seconds of one couple engaged in oral sex was followed by nine seconds of another couple in a Jacuzzi followed by six seconds of a housewife being drilled by a pizza deliveryman. And then a mailman. And then a plumber. It went on like this for what seemed an eternity.

Greenberg waited. And waited. And waited.

Perhaps the tape was stuck, he thought. Or perhaps this was just an unusually long trailer.

In any case, none of it was helping him get the ball across the finish line. Thankfully, there was no one else in the office but Greenberg and the statuesque blond receptionist/nurse/porn projector. So he did the unthinkable.

He got up from his chair, and with his sweatpants wrapped around his ankles, shuffled over to the door. He flipped the locks and cracked the door open a smidge.

Fill Up the Cup

Greenberg inched his face to the crevice.

"Excuse me."

No response.

Then louder, "Excuse me."

"Yes, Mr. Greenberg, is there a problem?"

"No problem. No problem whatsoever."

"Okay."

"But you can start now."

"I'm afraid I don't understand."

"I'm done with the trailers. You can start the movie now."

A long silent pause.

Followed by some giggling.

"Mr. Greenberg, that *is* the movie."

Now realizing his mistake, Larry slowly shut the door. But before he did, he heard the long leggy blond let out an involuntary cackle of laughter.

He tried returning to the mission, but it was not to be. Whether it was the nature of the short clips, the lack of any character or plot development, or the humiliating reaction from the sperm collection vixen, Larry would never say. He only knew the fight or flight response kicked in and he decided his best option was flight. He pulled his pants up and made a beeline for the exit door.

Fill Up the Cup

The next day, Greenberg had some explaining to do at the fertility doctor's office. But before she could start sassing him, he turned the tables on the doctor who majored, and minored, in labia.

"For eight months now I've been tugging at myself so we could fill up the turkey baster and for eight months we've come up with zilch. Why don't you tell us what's going on, Doc? Why are we still here? And why are there two of us when there should be three of us?"

Mrs. Greenberg was taken aback by his forcefulness. And not just a little bit turned on. The gynecologist was thunderstruck. Her tone was decidedly different.

"Well, the science of fertility has never been exact. And it never will be," she said, adding "perhaps it's time we take this to the next level."

Greenberg had no idea what that meant but seemed encouraged that his little burst of anger had elicited a reaction. And some respect.

"Ok," he said, "what's the next level?"

"Hormone shots. By enhancing the estrogen levels there's a good chance we can produce more eggs. And more eggs give us a greater probability of pregnancy. Perhaps even multiple pregnancy, like twins or triplets."

Greenberg was elated, "Damn, why didn't we do this before? We could get the whole family thing done in one fell swoop. A package deal, that's what I'm talking about."

"The shots are expensive," said the doctor, "$1,000 each."

Greenberg reeled at the price. And was even more deflated when he found out they were not reimbursed by his company's medical insurance.

"But there is a Plan B."

Fill Up the Cup

The doctor explained that while pharmaceutical companies in the US were charging exorbitant fees for the hormone shots, they were also available across the border. She told the Greenbergs that the same $1,000 shot sold at a pharmacy in Santa Monica was being sold in Tijuana for less than one-tenth the cost. They didn't even need a prescription. They could simply walk into a *pharmaceria*, lay down a C-note and walk away with the exact same medicine that was under tight FDA restrictions.

"That's great," said Greenberg, "we go down to Mexico, get the stuff, bring it back here to your office, and you'll inject my wife?"

"Uh, not quite."

Greenberg was not putting one-plus-one together.

"You're not allowed to bring this medicine back across the border. The injection will have to be administered while you are in Tijuana."

Greenberg scratched his chin, "So you would come with us down to Mexico? How does that work?"

"Oh no, I'm not going to Tijuana. I once bought a *serape* down there, thing was infested was fleas. Took me two months of soaking in Calamine lotion to get over that, I don't do Mexico."

"Am I hearing this right? You want us to go to Mexico buy the $1,000 hormone for $100 and then you want me to inject my wife with the shot?" asked Greenberg.

"That's the ticket."

She could tell from his reaction that was not the ticket.

"I'm not good with needles at all. And needles, in *Mexico*? In *Tijuana*? That's the trifecta of No, No and No."

Fill Up the Cup

"I don't know what else to tell you, Mr. Greenberg."

"Well, I have no similar loss of words – Good bye."

With that Larry Greenberg took hold of his wife's hand and guided her out of the doctor's office. As they rode down the elevator she noticed in him a fierce determination. It was as if he knew exactly what they were going to do. She had no idea. He was tight-lipped until they reached the car.

"Your days as a media sales rep are over."

"I can't quit my job, we need the money," said Mrs. Greenberg.

"We can get by on my salary. We'll tighten the belt, eat out less often and spend more time together at home. We don't need more money. We need less stress."

"Are you sure?"

"I've never been surer."

"OK, I'll give my two weeks notice tomorrow."

"We're not waiting until tomorrow. And we're not waiting another two weeks. I want you to quit working so we can start living. As a family."

He dropped her off at her office. Before he drove away, she grabbed him by the back of the head and kissed him like she hadn't kissed him in years. If he wasn't sure about this sudden surge of strong headedness, he was now.

As he got off the elevator at his office, Smithwick strolled up behind him and clutched him by the elbow.

Fill Up the Cup

"Where have you been?"

"Personal business."

"Well, here's some business you might want to take personally: Coughlin put the account up for review."

"That bitch!"

For six months Greenberg crisscrossed the country, sat in focus groups, and listened to her dull stories about the new drainage system she was installing at her summer home. He smiled when he didn't feel like smiling. He made small talk. And did his best to make her feel like there was nowhere else on Earth he'd rather be, when the complete opposite was true. He rewrote copy. He watered down ideas. He swallowed his pride until there was no pride left.

And he did all this while dry humping himself into little plastic cups with the hope of bringing a new Greenberg into this world to experience the same pleasure.

And this is how the world returns the favor?

"Jenkins wants to see you in his office."

"Probably to talk about how we were going to defend the account. This should be great," replied Greenberg.

Of course, that's not what Jenkins had in mind.

Twenty minutes later, Greenberg walked out of his office with a three-week severance check in his back pocket and a sinkhole in his stomach large enough for a small mammal. As he walked to the mailroom to get some empty cardboard boxes, his cell phone rang.

"I did it, honey. I quit. No notice. No questions. No nothing. It was great."

Fill Up the Cup

Greenberg bit his lip.

"I told you. Everything is going to work out," he assured her.

They made love that night.

And they made a baby, the old fashioned way. The way only two clueless, unemployed people with no foreseeable income and no future in advertising can.

A Few Rounds with Sonny Jaye

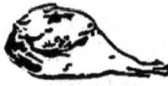

leg of mutton

A Few Rounds with Sonny Jaye

Sonny Jaye was a wiry son of a bitch.

He was lean and hard. But not in a way anyone would consider attractive. His body was twisted and asymmetrical. Fitness models had a six pack. Sonny had a five pack.

He was wound tight like the steel cables that hold up the Verrazano Bridge. If one of those thick, taut wires snapped, they would all unravel.

His unusually shaped body was the result of years of training in the gym. Sonny enjoyed boxing and spent all his waking hours in the ring. While the training had its effect on his physique, the hooks, the jabs and the uppercuts took its toll on his face.

His cheeks were unaligned. His forehead was bulbous. And his hairless skull resembled that of a Beluga whale. A blubberless, muscular and veiny Beluga whale.

Sonny Jaye was not an easy man to look at. Or even be around.

When he wasn't boxing he was plying his trade as a director of TV commercials. Not your run-of-the-mill local mattress store or car dealership commercials. Sonny had made it big time and was a bonafide A-lister, doing multi-million dollar productions. His Super Bowl spots made the Top Ten list year after year.

Not bad for an Irish kid who dropped out of university, left Dublin and spent countless years washing dishes at a shitty restaurant on Manhattan's 9th Ave. A restaurant that was considered shitty even by the low standards of Hell's Kitchen.

A Few Rounds with Sonny Jaye

The success, like the relentless left jabs from a skilled middleweight, went to his head.

Instead of saving money, Sonny spent it. He bought houses he never lived in. He bought cars he never drove. And he wore clothes that were more befitting a Harlem pimp and less a man who regularly found himself conducting business transactions with the CEO's of Fortune 500 companies.

His appearance was odd. And his behavior was even odder.

Despite his pugilistic skills, he surrounded himself with a phalanx of beefy bodyguards. He would experiment with his own diets. For an entire month he consumed nothing but nonfat chocolate milk and celery sticks. He swore off the use of telephones. Not because he developed a fear of germs or anything that seemed remotely rational, he just didn't like telephones.

Despite his eccentricities, or perhaps because of them, creative people in the advertising community desperately wanted to work with the great Sonny Jaye.

Maybe, they thought, his magic would rub off on their ideas. Or he'd improve work that had no business being in production. One solid spot from Sonny Jaye could make or break a career.

The famous Talking Cockroach campaign vaulted a junior team out of London to Associate Creative Directors at Wieden & Kennedy's Portland office.

Witness the success of the Black Belt Grandma spot. A year ago, two kids who were doing banner ads managed to get one TV spot made with Sonny and now they're running the JWT/Anchorage office.

And then there were the two Creative Directors, in their mid-40's, who were slowly being shown the door despite their new tattoos and stylish Trilby hats. They teamed up with Mr. Jaye to make a long form spot about a solar-powered coffee grinder.

It went viral. The greying pair left advertising and signed a three-year development deal with Disney.

These are the stories that made Sonny Jaye an industry legend. But there were other stories as well. His lavish spending had outpaced his obscene income earning. As a result, Sonny had become less discerning about the jobs he agreed to accept as long as he could keep his creditors at bay.

It was under these circumstances that art director Don Curley and copywriter Jeff Silver found themselves seated in a production office conference room across the table from the iconic Sonny Jaye.

As Sonny was gently laying his feathered wide brim Stetson on the mahogany table, Silver took the opportunity to break the ice.

"We're big fans of your work and we wanted to let you know what an..."

Sonny interrupted.

"Yeah, I don't do the small talk thing. Let's go over the storyboards and get on with it."

Silver reached behind his seat and grabbed the first foamcore board. He laid it flat on the table so Sonny could give it a good look and then started explaining the concept.

"In this first spot, we open at a typical middle class home. The husband is very excited about an upcoming delivery."

A cell phone started ringing. Sonny reached into the pocket of his double-breasted, bright yellow blazer and pulled out the culprit.

A Few Rounds with Sonny Jaye

"Ah, the rumors aren't true," Curley thought. Sonny handed the phone to a curvaceous assistant to his right. She answered the phone and began whispering in Sonny's ear.

"The rumors are true," Curley thought again.

It went back and forth, the dialogue punctuated by several terse replies.

"Tell him no."

"That's not what I want."

"Because I said so, that's why."

And then, when he could contain himself no longer, Sonny grabbed the phone from his production assistant and stormed off into the corner.

"Here's the deal. I don't want a shepherd that's a quarter wolf or half wolf. I want a wolf wolf. And if they don't agree to one, I'm not doing the shoot. Cause it'll be shiite," his Irish accent was getting thicker, "and I don't do shiiite!"

Curley, Silver and the entire agency team wondered what they had got themselves into.

They arrived in Chatsworth on a cool April morning. Normally, when neighbors in Chatsworth see production trucks hijacking the parking spots and setting up the catering tables, they know exactly what to expect. But today was different.

The cast, the crew, the caterers, the retired motorcycle cops who would tell stories of the glory days, were all there for a Sonny Jaye masterpiece.

A Few Rounds with Sonny Jaye

Sonny was inexplicably chipper. Curley and Silver thought he was bipolar. Or had a pharmaceutical connection worth knowing about.

"Good morning, mates. A fine day to put some magic on film, don't you say?"

"If only," Curley thought. His seven-year-old daughter just got fitted for orthodontia. With the promise of many more years of expensive dental work to come. A great campaign, a promotion and a raise would be just the tonic he needed to defray the outrageous cost.

Silver, too, needed a home run. His older brother was a successful corporate litigator in Washington, DC. And his younger sister was on her way to a PhD in Organic Chemistry.

His failure to produce anything worthwhile, let alone visible, had become a favorite topic of his disappointed father at family get-togethers. The old man could not understand Silver's decision to pursue a career in advertising. Nor how it merited an expensive four year education at Stanford.

A production assistant came by with a tray of drinks for Sonny and the agency creatives.

"Banana/kale/Greek yogurt smoothie?"

As the crew was duct taping marks for the actors and rearranging furniture in the living room of the modest Chatsworth home, Curley was troubled by the lack of lighting equipment. He murmured something to Silver, who suggested he question Sonny.

"I'm not a big believer in that," said Sonny.

"Natural performances require natural lighting. You see these other directors bring in the Fisher Light Box and the 10K's and all their fancy screens and filters. It's all rubbish. It's all for show. Completely unnecessary. I've got the sun and that's plenty."

Curley checked the monitor and wasn't happy with the lighting fill on the lead actress.

"You think it's too dark?" Sonny replied, "We'll open some windows. We'll open doors. Hell, I've got a crew here that's handy with a Sawzall, we'll cut a hole in the roof. We'll patch it up afterwards. We've done it before."

Curley looked at Sonny's executive producer who was nodding, silently.

"Lighting packages? Those are for amateurs."

A Ford F250 monster truck pulled into the driveway. Behind it was an open flatbed trailer. Penned in the trailer was a very pink, very large 600 pound pig. The pig, seemingly unaware that he had made a 50 mile trip from Ojai to Chatsworth and had arrived on a film set, was chewing on whatever it is they give to pigs before going for a 50 mile ride.

Sonny dropped everything to run outside and pet the pig.

The executive producer, anticipating the response of most non-bipolar people, turned to Curley and Silver, shrugged and simply offered, "Don't ask."

If they were apprehensive before the camera started rolling, the words "speed" and "action" did little to comfort them. This is typically the moment when ad agency art directors and copywriters know whether they have made a wise directorial decision or not. It was increasingly apparent that Curley and Silver had erred. Big time.

Some directors like to bark at actors, screaming at the top of their lungs even offering line readings.

"Do it like this. No, not like that. Like this."

Others are more hands off and allow the players to play, improvise and find their characters.

And still others prefer a shotgun approach, shooting each scene small, bigger and broad, giving the storytellers plenty of options in the edit bay.

Sonny employed none of these tried and true methods. In addition to not bringing any lighting equipment to shoot, he brought little in the way of ideas. He simply let the camera roll. And roll. And roll.

He never yelled "cut" and he never offered anything in the way of direction. At the end of every scene, with the camera still rolling, he'd simply offer, "Let's take it again from the top."

By day's end, he had burned through 15,000 feet of film. He also burned through an ensemble of frustrated actors who are normally happy to be hired for any job, but who were markedly upset they had accepted this one. As they left the set they made a point of telling Curley and Silver they'd prefer taking sock inventory at The Gap than working with this pig-petting, pretentious asshole ever again.

The second day of production brought the cast and crew to the Inland Empire. The Happy Time Hot Tub Company had agreed to rent out their facilities for a day of filming on the warehouse floor.

Breakfast burritos were eaten. Asparagus/lemon/sour cream smoothies were sucked through straws. Lighting paraphernalia was not set up. And for no apparent reason, a 600 pound sunburnt pig was shanghaied out to Riverside, CA.

Maybe it was the new setting. Maybe it was the new actors. Maybe it was because Sonny's executive producer had a few course-correcting words with him prior to the shoot, but the day's shooting had been going remarkably better.

This put Curley and Silver at ease. And it made their client, a dotcom company teetering on the edge of financial disaster, a little more hopeful about the agency's marketing plan.

They made it to lunchtime without a hitch. Sonny had the good grace to sit with Curley and Silver and their nervous client. Over delicious tri-tip sandwiches, Israeli couscous and fire-roasted vegetables they even exchanged small talk.

Sonny put out a vague, half-hearted invitation for all of them to get together at his villa in the Maldives. He talked about the possibility of shooting a feature film with Channing Tatum. And he let them know that the craft service lunch they were all enjoying came from the skilled hands of his personal chef, Raoul Garcia, who travelled the globe with Sonny, catering all his meals.

"I love this man," said Sonny.

Then, loud enough so Raoul could hear him in the food truck, he shouted in butchered Spanish, "Muchas gracias, Raoul. Es mucho excellente."

"*Pinche tu madre*," Raoul muttered to himself.

The shooting resumed and the mood remained light, courteous and professional. They were in the homestretch now.

The last scene needed to complete the story for the commercial involved an inattentive hot tub manufacturer who ignores the phone call of an irate customer. The actor had been rehearsing and was perfect for the part. The set had been cleared. The warehouse doors had been locked so that there would be no interruptions.

Sonny was about to call "action" when suddenly Silver brought up what should have been a minor issue.

"Can we move the phone?"

A Few Rounds with Sonny Jaye

"Move it? Move it where?" replied Sonny.

"Anywhere, just not so close to the guy. We need the phone answering machine to take the call."

"Why can't the phone be right next to him? He just chooses to ignore it," said Sonny.

"Most people who are standing next to a ringing phone will pick it up."

"Well, he doesn't." Sonny stood his ground.

Silver got up from his seat in the video village and came over to talk more discreetly with the director.

"I don't want this to be a thing. Can we just move the phone?" he whispered.

"We can. But I'm not," said Sonny.

"What?"

"Oh, and it's a thing," added Sonny.

At this point you could hear 75 production crew members, who had seen the volatile Sonny Jaye movie before, take a collective breath.

"You don't like where the phone is. I'm going to tell you what I don't like."

Oh shit, thought Silver.

" I don't like pissant art directors..."

"I'm a copywriter."

A Few Rounds with Sonny Jaye

"I don't like pissant copywriters stepping onto my set telling me my business. Do I barge into your office and tell you to change incredible to remarkable?"

"I wouldn't use either of those words."

"Do I stand over your shoulder while you're typing and tell you to lose the ellipses because I can't stand ellipses?"

"I don't use ellipses, either."

"Do I fuckin' fuck with you? You fuckin' fuckwit?"

Silver had had enough.

He stood toe to toe with Sonny, jutted out his jaw and said, "What is your deal?"

Sonny smiled. And Silver couldn't help noticing the vein that ran up and down Sonny's neck had tripled in width.

"You want to know my deal? I'll show you my deal."

Sonny, who could have laid Silver out with a well-rehearsed left cross, whirled back and spotted a white wooden folding chair that had been used by the crew at lunchtime. He grabbed the sturdy chair with both hands and wheeled it back over his head.

The crew, many of them with iPhones in their hands, inhaled again.

He swung the chair in a wild arc, coming down on the warehouse floor with all 153 pounds of his wiry might. A seven-inch section of the left leg ricocheted off the hard cement and nearly caught a planner in the shin.

With the speed of a trained welterweight, he brought the chair back over his head while people were still reeling from the first blow.

A Few Rounds with Sonny Jaye

The floor gave no quarter. The cross slats that supported the legs splintered off and flew in all directions.

Sonny had made his point. But while there was still a recognizable chair in his hands, he wanted to leave no room for error.

He smashed the chair down a third time.

A fourth time.

A fifth time.

A sixth time.

A seventh time.

It went on for an eternity. And witnesses described the moment as surreal. As if, despite the lightning quick violence, it was all happening in slow motion.

When the chair was gone and all that remained was a scattered pile of shards and sawdust, so was Sonny. He dropped the last piece of wood left in his hand like a rapper dropping the mic to signify an uncontested victory. He walked away from the dramatic demolition and left the warehouse building.

"Holy Mother of God!" said the sound guy to the key grip. Adding, "I've never seen anything like that."

Indeed nobody, veterans from both the production side and agency side of the business, no strangers to hot temperament, had ever seen anyone go that ballistic. With the exception of the hum from the Happy Time KZ 9000™ floor model hot tub with the patented Soothamatic jets, there wasn't a sound in the warehouse.

Glub, glub, glub, hmmmmm, glub, glub, glub, hmmmmm.

Minutes later, Sonny Jaye re-entered the building. And acted as if nothing had transpired. Nothing at all.

"Let's move those C-Stands. Let's move the camera over here. And, in accordance with the requests from our new director (looking towards Silver), let's put the phone over here."

Production assistants snapped out of their daze and began to scurry around. But Silver would have none of that.

"Whoa. What do you think you're doing?"

"We're getting the last shot for the spot, mate."

"No. No, we're not."

"Come again?"

"We're not shooting one more frame of film until you explain yourself and apologize to everyone on this production for your brutish, uncalled for, violent and outrageous behavior," said Silver. Adding, "Everybody. Just. Stop."

"What? Oh that, mate? Is was a bit of show."

"A show?"

"Performance theater. I know plenty of people who'd pay a few shillings to see something that good on Piccadilly Circus. Know what I mean, guvnor?"

"No. I don't know what you mean, guvnor."

"Ease up there, pal. You've been around the block, you know the deal, it's all part of the show."

A Few Rounds with Sonny Jaye

"I don't know what show you're talking about. What I do know is that human beings don't treat other human beings like that. They have disagreements and they find ways to work out those disagreements. What they don't do is go full on *Incredible Hulk* and start busting up the furniture."

Sonny replied, "I heard that on the set of *2001, A Space Odyssey*, Kubrick got so upset with an actor who couldn't remember his lines that he went on a spectacular tirade, rampaged through the set and put his foot through Uranus."

"OK, three things. Three very important things," interrupted Silver, "you're not Stanley Kubrick. Second, we're not on a set shooting a piece of cinema. Third, as if needs to be repeated, you're not Stanley Fuckin' Kubrick."

Sonny looked around and found he could not fault Silver for his logic.

"You are a washed up, talentless hack directing a TV commercial on a set, in a warehouse, in the seedy outskirts of Riverside, California, for a dotcom company that probably won't see a second round of VC funding."

Sonny smirked. The financially strapped client grimaced.

Silver added, "I'll say it again, we're not shooting one more frame of film until you apologize."

"That's not happening," said Sonny.

"Then neither is this spot," replied Silver.

He turned to the crew and raised his right hand in a slashing motion under his own throat. The production team knew exactly where their bread was being buttered. They got paid by the client and the ad agency. And not by Sonny Jaye.

Generators wound down and the team began the long process of breaking the set.

A week later, Curley and Silver found themselves in the bay with their favorite editor, Frank Shambaugh. Frank looked at the film and was not very hopeful. Half the footage was underexposed. He couldn't do a montage sequence. There wasn't a cross fade or a fancy star wipe that could save them now. They had an unmitigated disaster on their hands.

This is the end they thought. The client is going to freak. The agency is going to cut them loose. And they'll ride out the rest of their careers writing Pharma spots for cholesterol lowering potions, vaginal meshes and COPD mucus remedies.

"I'd like to tear that Irishman a new arsehole," said Curley.

Shambaugh scratched his bearded chin.

He pecked away on the keyboard of his oversized Mac and called the guys over to look at something. It was a YouTube video titled, *The Making of a Cadillac Car Commercial.*

Curley and Silver yawned.

"These are the worst navel-gazing experiences ever put on film."

"Look it has 174 views on YouTube. Who wants to watch the sausage being made? Now you set that sausage factory on fire and then you might have something to crow about."

Frank looked at his two colleagues as if to say, "Exactly."

They called the production company. Got in touch with every crew member. And collected all the iPhone clips of the colossal Sonny Jaye meltdown. The screaming. The fighting. The chair busting. They even managed to get some shots of the 600 pound pig catching a mid-afternoon nap.

They documented the whole fiasco in a short three minute film titled, *The Un-Making of a TV Commercial.*

It was the look behind the curtain that was finally worth looking at.

In two weeks time, *The Un-Making of a TV Commercial* had amassed more than eight million hits on YouTube.

Trade magazines were lining up at the door to interview Curley and Silver. They did the circuit of morning shows, tabloid shows and late night talk shows. And even though their client didn't get the TV commercials they had been promised, they got something more valuable – free press.

$12 million worth of free press. And with that came their precious second round of VC funding. Followed by a third. And an IPO.

Channing Tatum's people backed out of the pending movie deal. And Sonny never made a feature film.

He was no longer an A-list director. He wasn't even a B or C. The last anyone had seen from Sonny Jaye, he was bidding on a package of spots for an off-brand of Slovenian erectile dysfunction pills.

The 33rd Prawn

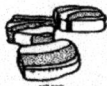

sushi prawn

Hiko Yamamoto had a vocabulary of 300 English words. Rarely were any of those words successfully strung together into a meaningful phrase. There just wasn't much call for "umbrella bathroom" or "cheeseburger pencil."

He was, however, familiar with the concept of "no." As well as the notion of "good," and spared no opportunity to pair the two.

Despite his third grade command of the language and his even more childlike understanding of American culture, Hiko Yamamoto was named the Chief Marketing Officer for the Lexus Motor Company headquartered in Torrance, California. His appointment caught many off guard. And gave rise to increased tension in the laid back Southern California offices, which often found itself at odds with their overlords on the other side of the Pacific.

Yamamoto was not the first English-deficient senior ranking executive Japan had sent over to show the Americans how it's done. And his predecessors ~ stony robotic men ~ were rarely invited over for backyard BBQ's or added to any of the Torrance local's Christmas card list.

His appointment came complements of the Lexus Round Robin Executive Grooming System. The program might not have a very official sounding name but the premise was solid. At least, on paper.

Every three years, the organization would turn itself over. That is, executives would rotate from one field of professional expertise to the next. Design guys would move over to sales. Manufacturing people would take a crack at service. And finance pros would go into marketing. The cross pollination would not be limited by national boundaries. Lexus executives often found themselves shipped to China, Malaysia, England and, of course, the US.

The goal was to develop well-rounded employees who could bring a wealth of experience to any business challenge. It would also reduce the occurrence of executive burnout, which had become very common; as common as a *gaijin* walking into a Kyoto sushi bar, ordering the California Roll, and asking for a fork.

Upper brass at Lexus had also told themselves it was a way to stay true to their slogan, "The Relentless Pursuit of Perfection." It meant not just producing excellent automobiles that could go head to head with their German competitors, it meant producing excellent salary men and women who could succeed in any area.

The automotive press across the pond was not so optimistic.

At an industry presser in Long Beach they peppered Yamamoto with questions. About his credentials. About his understanding of American culture. And how he planned to navigate the nuanced world of luxury automobile marketing, a sector worth more than $5 billion.

The questions were fielded by his fawning underling and translated for Yamamoto. What his answers lacked in substance, they more than made up for in brevity.

"Yes."

"No."

He also sprinkled in some aphorisms, knowing American journalists – the laziest people on Earth – were fond of sound bites.

"The greatest risk is not taking one."

"You must try. Or hate yourself for not trying."

The 33rd Prawn

"There are two ways a man can learn: university and adversity."

Mike Cronin threw down his copy of *Car & Driver* and mumbled to no one in particular, "Oh great, another graduate from the School of Fortune Cookie Management."

Cronin was Yamamoto's stateside counterpart and had been working at Lexus for the past 12 years. He knew the next three years under Yamamoto's thumb would test his fortitude. He had outlasted Takahashi, Yakuma and Kishiyama, and through perseverance, resiliency, and vast quantities of Tanqueray and Tonic, he knew he would survive this.

Besides, what choice did he have?

He and his wife had just enrolled their twins at a private school. The tile counter in the kitchen had just been remodeled with inordinately expensive soapstone. And the bathroom downstairs has been regularly burping back an ugly cocktail of raw sewage, meaning the pipe to the street would have to be fully trenched out and replaced, an operation that would set his portfolio back to 2009.

His rise through the corporate ranks had been markedly different than Yamamoto's.

Cronin played college football for the Iowa Hawkeyes. His tenacity at right tackle earned him a spot in the NFL, two promising seasons with the Cincinnati Bengals. While battling their cross-state rivals, the Cleveland Browns, Cronin was chop blocked by a desperate left guard and tore his ACL. He was sidelined for five months. The ACL never healed properly and Cronin's career path was sent in another direction.

Another retired Pro Bowler had opened a car dealership and was happy to take Mike on as an apprentice salesman.

The 33rd Prawn

He wasn't an apprentice for very long. Customers took an immediate liking to Cronin's teddy bear quality. Despite his massive size, six-foot four-inches tall and tipping the scales at 320 pounds, on a good day, he was soft spoken, gentle and unassuming.

It was a winning combination if there ever was one. Plus, with every sale he'd hand out a signed photograph as well as a signed regulation NFL football. Car buyers lined up to give Cronin their money.

He didn't remain at any position for very long. To the dismay of his colleagues Cronin won all the salesman contests. He went to Aruba on so many paid vacations, he was known to the locals and became an excellent limbo dancer. To make him ineligible for the monthly challenges, the other salesman voted to have Mike Cronin promoted and made District Sales Manager.

Soon after, he was made Regional Sales Manager. And soon after that he was called west, to begin work at the corporate office. The pace never slowed down and success followed Mike wherever he went.

Until there was no higher to go.

As the top American executive of Lexus North America it was his responsibility to work side by side with Mr. Yamamoto. At least that's how it was described to him in the memo from Japan. The reality was he would work under the thumb of Yamamoto, who had the bedside manner of Colonel Saito from *Bridge Over the River Kwai*.

It wasn't long before workers at the Torrance office starting calling Yamamoto, behind his back, Colonel, or Saito.

At Shaughnessey's Irish Tavern, across the street from headquarters, many a late night ended with drunken, miserable employees griping about their situations and mocking their new imperial taskmaster.

"The bridge must be built. The bridge must be built."

The 33rd Prawn

The Yamamoto/Cronin honeymoon did not last long. It couldn't. There were three new vehicles to launch and there was no time for niceties. Besides, honeymoon periods are usually born of the desire to get along. To be friendly. To make a good impression.

Yamamoto wasn't interested in any of that.

Barely a week into his position, he asked to see the advertising campaign for the new mid sized SUV.

"Great news on that front, Mr. Yamamoto, the team from the ad agency is already on a plane to Canada to begin filming that commercial on Wednesday," said Cronin.

The translator nervously put the words into Japanese.

"No."

"Uh, no?" Mike replied, "The team is already in route. The locations have been scouted. The cast had been assembled. And the check to the production company had already been cut."

None of that made any sense. And not because the words were in English.

The translator looked at Cronin as if to say, "Do you really want me to tell him that?"

He didn't have to answer. Yamamoto rattled off a long diatribe, in Japanese, punctuated by shouting and some guttural noises no one in the Torrance office had ever heard before.

The translator sprung the nightmare scenario on Cronin.

Cancel the shoot.

Bring the team back.

The 33rd Prawn

Start over.

Cronin bit down hard on the inside of his cheek. His assistant ran from the room to make the necessary phone calls and stop the financial bleeding. But she ran too soon, because the coal raking was not yet complete. In addition to killing the approved work, which had instantaneously become worthless old work, Yamamoto stated in no uncertain terms, that he wanted to see new work in two days.

"Two days?" Cronin stammered. "That's impossible. It'll take one day just to fly the creative team back home. And they're going to be crushed. I can't ask them..."

He stopped mid-sentence, realizing that logic had not been invited to this particular meeting.

"What's the new strategy, Mr. Yamamoto?"

"Luxury," Yamamoto replied.

"Anything more?" the translator asked.

"Luxury."

Yamamoto grabbed his wire frame glasses and left the room, knowing full well in two days he'd be in the same room judging new work presented to him by smiling American ad people who would gladly do his bidding.

"The bridge must be built."

Thanks to his many years playing football, Cronin understood the mechanics of the two-minute drill. He told the brass at the ad agency to get all hands on deck. There was no time to fret about the cart suddenly being upended. He told his finance people that money was no object and instructed the agency to hire freelancers, work around the clock and bring ideas that will stop the leak in the dam.

Cronin decided he would go with the all-out blitz. Since he had no idea what Yamamoto liked or didn't like, get or didn't get, he opted for quantity, with the hope that there would be some glimmer of quality.

Two days later, a dozen art directors and copywriters sat outside the mahogany-paneled conference room at Lexus headquarters. Six teams had each prepared three storyboards. A total of 18 separate ideas would be presented for Mr. Yamamoto's consideration.

Before the teams entered the room to face the dragon, they were given some quick rules of engagement.

"Do not under any circumstances attempt to shake hands with Mr. Yamamoto."

"Do not look Mr. Yamamoto directly in the eyes. Avert your stare."

"And finally, do not attempt to defend your work or editorialize. Once you are done presenting, simply bow and leave the room."

The parade began.

The first team had only been at the agency for eight months. They were still wet behind the ears. Nobody expected them to hit it out of the park. So when Yamamoto barely grunted at their ideas, no one was very surprised.

They were merely the warm up act. Their purpose was to grease the skids. To demonstrate how the agency had pulled out all the stops and would tirelessly work to please Mr. Yamamoto.

Surely, Cronin thought, teams two, three and four would have better luck.

The grunting had now been replaced with something that resembled speaking. And impossibly, Yamamoto's mood had turned from sour to sourer.

"...and then the logo comes up over the car and we fade to black."

"ダメません," said Yamamoto.

"No good," his translator translated.

Idea number 12.

"ダメません," said Yamamoto.

"No good," his translator translated.

Idea number 13.

"ダメません," said Yamamoto.

"No good," his translator translated.

Idea number 14.

"ダメません," said Yamamoto.

"No good," his translator translated.

Idea number 15.

"ダメません," said Yamamoto.

Cronin stopped the translator, "No good, I get it."

The last team entered the room. These were seasoned veterans who had won all kinds of awards and who were actively being recruited by several high profile agencies. Cronin knew they had always delivered and were confident they had cracked this nut.

He also knew the reflexive "no good" was of no value, particularly if the teams needed to return to the drawing board. A fate that looked more likely than ever. Cronin needed Yamamoto to explain why an idea was "no good."

Yamamoto was slow to respond to Idea #16. A glimmer of hope perhaps. He reached across the table and carefully followed the progression of illustrations on the storyboard. He put the board down and cleared his throat.

"ダメません," said Yamamoto.

"Why?" Cronin interjected, "Why don't you like it?"

The translator obliged and Yamamoto rattled off a few dozen animated words of Japanese.

"Mr. Yamamoto likes this idea very much. He says it has many fine qualities. And believes could be very successful," said the translator.

Cronin felt his shoulders loosen.

"But commercial is no good."

"Huh?" said Cronin.

"We see here in frame four, car makes left turn," said the translator.

Cronin picked up the storyboard to confirm that minor point.

"Yes, yes, the car makes a left turn, I see it," offered Cronin.

"Left turn is considered very unprofessional."

"Wait, what? A left turn is un...professional?" said a stunned Cronin. "This is just a storyboard. We'll change it to a right turn."

"ダメません," barked Yamamoto.

The last two ideas met a similar fate. One was no good because there was a woman driving the vehicle, this seemed important since the appeal of a mid sized SUV was to women. Nevertheless, it didn't appeal to Mr. Yamamoto. And the last idea went down in flames because the car in the storyboard was dark green. And, as Cronin was to discover, dark green is not luxurious.

"Dark green is very ruxurious," Cronin so wanted to scream, but wisely nodded and remained silent.

It was the worst creative presentation Cronin ever had the misfortune to witness.

The process, not unlike the Bataan Death March, went on for months. Until Yamamoto had *Frankensteined* a commercial, taking pieces from one campaign and stitching them together with pieces from another campaign, with no regard for logic or nuance.

It was painful, irrational and costly. Over the course of the next three months, the ad agency reporting to Yamamoto and Lexus had lost half its creative department.

When the commercial was complete, no one, other than Yamamoto, wanted to have their name associated with the work. During post-production, when credits are assigned to the commercial for record-keeping purposes or award show entries, the ad agency people stole a page from the playbook of their movie brethren. Directors, writers and producers not wanting to be associated with Hollywood stinkers would often replace their names with that of a fictional character named Alan Smithee.

The 33rd Prawn

In the advertising community there was no Alan Smithee, but there was E. Vincent Cummings a despised creative director that many had toiled under and whose lack of talent was only surpassed by his grating pomposity. It was a meaningless gesture but it gave those touched by this nightmare a small sense of retribution.

Creative Director: E. Vincent Cummings

Copywriter: E. Vincent Cummings

Art Director: E. Vincent Cummings

Client: Hiko Yamamoto

Cronin would sit in his office for hours watching the spot over and over again. Perhaps his instincts and the instincts of every other American on staff were wrong. It had happened before. Maybe Yamamoto and his unusual non-linear thinking were onto something. It could have been a cultural difference of opinion, East vs. West. Cronin was open-minded and thoughtful enough to entertain that notion.

He watched the spot one more time.

He was right. It was shit.

Before the commercial would air on national TV, it was customary to unveil it before a national gathering of the top dealers. It was important to get their buy-in and galvanize the folks who would be most responsible for moving the sheet metal.

Yamamoto's translator, a man of many talents, arranged for the confab at the Mandalay Bay Hotel in Las Vegas. The catering department at the Mandalay had been told to spare no expense. The vegetables were to be fresh. The bread was to be baked that day. The chocolate was to be flown in from Switzerland. It was Yamamoto's first time to meet and greet the dealers and he wanted, and expected, everything to be on point.

A rolling bar had been set outside the hallway of the Roosevelt Banquet room. Here, the oily men and women who closed the deals and persuaded unknowing customers to spring for useless undercoat protection and worthless credit insurance, gathered, cajoled and shared war stories.

While they drank enough whiskey to put the state of Kentucky on Defcon 2, Yamamoto quietly slipped into the large banquet room where final preparations were being made.

The roast beef was carved to perfection.

The assorted cheeses were meticulously cubed.

And the jumbo prawns were arranged on circular platters as if Fibonacci himself had supervised the operation.

Everything was just right.

Almost.

Yamamoto shouted so loud the chandeliers were rattling. The translator was startled. And Cronin muttered to himself, "Here we go."

The yelling and screaming had reached unprecedented levels. And Cronin wondered, what could possibly set off such a tantrum.

The translator did his best to bring the simmering down. Then whisked Cronin off to the side.

"There is a problem with the prawns."

"Oh, for a minute I thought it was something important," replied Cronin.

"This *is* important. Mr. Yamamoto was under the impression that each circular serving platter would have 33 prawns. The last platter on the table only has 32."

"OK, " said Cronin, still wondering what the commotion was all about. "So it has 32 prawns, who's counting?"

"Mr. Yamamoto is counting," said the translator.

"Tell Mr. Yamamoto it's a prawn, no one gives a hoot whether there's 32 or 33 shrimp on the god-damned platt...," Cronin stopped himself, anticipating the illogical reaction.

"It is a matter of symmetry," the translator tried to explain. Adding, "Very, very important."

Cronin rolled his eyes, having heard the symmetry sermon many times over the past few painful months. This was not the time or the place for another condescending lecture on Asian sensibilities.

"Tell the catering manager to get another shrimp up here pronto," snapped Cronin.

"I'm told they do not have any more prawns."

"Have somebody run up the street to Caesar's or The Excalibur. We're on the Las Vegas strip for Christ's sake. You're telling me we can't find a frikkin' jumbo shrimp?"

The 20-minute delay turned into a 40-minute delay.

And 200 drunken car dealers turned into an impatient horde, who wanted to see the commercials, chow down on some red meat and hit the gentlemen's clubs with a thick wad of tens and twenties in their pockets. The Cialis and Viagra were kicking in. And a middle-aged erection is a terrible thing to waste.

Cronin wanted to tell Yamamoto this was not the way to wins hearts and minds. But he also knew that any pleading on his part would be met with the thousand-yard stare.

"The bridge must be built."

Cronin turned on the charm and worked the room like the bride at an Italian wedding. At the risk of overpromising, he assured each dealer that the wait would be worth it. Then he spotted Ned Clauson pawing a waitress and making his way to the bar. He knew Ned from his college football playing days.

Clauson liked his liquor. The liquor didn't always return the favor. One minute he could be jovial and the funniest guy on Earth. But one Wild Turkey too many and the joking could become jabbing. Punch lines replaced by punches. With Clauson, chaos, sometimes criminal, was never out of the question.

Tonight, his fuse was even shorter. His dealership in Dayton, Ohio, was failing miserably. Between the lingering effects of the recession and the disappearance of Rust Belt revenue, Clauson was barely keeping his head above water. Earlier in the day, at the crustacean-less breakfast, he confided to Cronin that this commercial and the launch of this new SUV was his last hope.

Clauson stumbled up to the bar. Again. As the bartender filled another highball glass with cracked ice, Cronin turned to the translator.

"I need to get Clauson in and out of here in a hurry. If he's not at the Crazy Horse with two jasmine-scented strippers named Candy and Destiny sprawled across his lap, we're gonna need Mandalay Bay's biggest, baddest bruisers down here to break things up."

The 33rd Prawn

The catering manager, still huffing and puffing, ran up to Cronin with some goods news.

"We found a shrimp."

"Excellent," said Cronin, "Where is it?"

"At Harrah's."

"Get it."

"Harrah's in Laughlin. I can have it flown up here in an hour and half."

Cronin looked over at Clauson, who was now chiding the bartender, "Stop Jewing down the drinks!"

"We don't have an hour and a half," said Cronin.

The translator did not stick around for the play by play. He ran inside the banquet hall and took matters into his own hands.

Three minutes later, the quick-thinking translator ushered Yamamoto in for a final inspection of the banquet room.

Once satisfied, the doors swung open and the Lexus Dealers of America entered the Roosevelt Hall, where amongst the beautiful settings they found perfectly arranged platters, each featuring the exact same number of jumbo prawns.

"I don't understand," said Cronin.

"When it became apparent that we would never secure the 33rd prawn, I did the next best thing and asked the catering staff to remove a shrimp from each of the other platters."

"So they each had 32!" said Cronin, "That's genius, Keiji (addressing the translator by name for the first time in four months), genius."

Ned Clauson got some grub in his belly, dinner went off without a hitch and Mr. Yamamoto unveiled his first US made commercial, which was given a tepid reception by the inebriated dealership body.

The American public was not quite so forgiving. The launch of the luxury mid-size SUV failed miserably.

The press dubbed it the worst television commercial ever made. When it debuted on Agency Spy, the industry's favorite online gossip site, it broke all records for snarky comments, reaching unprecedented levels and crashing the server for three consecutive days.

With little fanfare, Mr. Yamamoto was summoned back to Japan.

The Round Robin Executive Program also came to an abrupt halt. In fact, when the brass gathered to assess the damage and act accordingly, they broke rank with the past and for the first time ever sought the advice of their Yankee colleagues for the selection of Mr. Yamamoto's U.S. replacement.

Cronin responded immediately, saying he had the perfect candidate who spoke both languages, understood the dynamics of the corporate relationship with dealers and had an uncanny ability to think outside the box.

Within a week of Yamamoto's departure, his translator Keiji Toyama was named the new CEO of Lexus North America. He thanked Cronin, his colleague, and now, new partner for all that he had done on his behalf.

"Symmetry, Mr. Toyama, it's all about the symmetry."

Himmelfarb Finds His Mojo

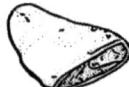

Parma ham

Himmelfarb Finds His Mojo

"This is not your best work."

Himmelfarb took the criticism with great aplomb. At least on the surface. He'd been in advertising for quite some time and knew all the little motivational tricks employed by Creative Directors. And this new one, Rogozinski, brought in from Chicago's hottest ad agency – an oxymoron as far as Himmelfarb was concerned – was no different.

"Why don't you and your partner take another stab at it," added Rogozinski.

Well, of course he and his partner were going to take another stab at it. They were in the multiple stabbing business. That's what creative teams did these days. They got briefed at 10 A.M. on a Monday and were expected to show work by 4 P.M. on Monday – the same Monday.

Everything put on paper was simply a stab in the dark. There was never any guidance. Or insight. Or time to stew on an idea, let it simmer, percolate and morph into something amazing.

There were only overbearing clients with overbearing timelines. If Internet pages were going to be taken over with flashy graphics and scroll-interrupting mechanisms that people love so much, agencies had to move fast.

Faster than fast. A demanding public awaits their online advertising, brand engagement units, and scalable individualized ecosystems.

"Let's see where you guys are at eight tonight?" shot Rogozinski, as he was off to review more work from other teams working on even shorter deadlines.

Himmelfarb Finds His Mojo

Eight? Himmelfarb thought, by that time I should be home, eating with my family and comparing notes on their crappy day.

With his new boss clearly out of sight, Himmelfarb and his art director skulked away.

"Sure, why don't we reconvene in five and a half hours and see if we've made any progress repositioning this billion dollar global brand for the next decade," said the frustrated copywriter.

Tris, his stoic partner, was a woman not given to griping. She trailed behind him. She knew through years of experience that is was best to let him vent. In many ways, having creative work killed was like going through the grieving process. Initially there's denial, followed by anger, resentment, acceptance and healing.

Of course, it was also her work, but she didn't take it as a personal attack. She did what Himmelfarb could not: she shrugged her shoulders and moved on.

Now, on these condensed deadlines, it would take Himmelfarb a good 45 minutes to get through all the phases. When he did, Tris took the opportunity to say something she had been thinking for quite some time.

"I didn't want to say anything, but I have to."

"What's up?"

"Rogozinski could be right."

"Right how?"

"I don't know how to put this."

"Just put it. Blurt it out," said Himmelfarb.

Himmelfarb Finds His Mojo

"You're overthinking this stuff."

"Overthinking?"

"You said to blurt it out. I'm blurting," Tris countered.

"How am I overthinking?"

"You're talking at people instead of with them. I don't know how else to put it. There's this precious quality to your language. Save that for your screenplay. This is advertising. We're shilling shit to the masses and trying to move the merchandise."

"Are you saying I'm snobby?"

"When was the last time you went East of La Cienega?" she asked.

"Uhhhh. I went to New York last month."

"Did you land in Newark?"

"Yup."

"Did you visit your high school pals in Hackensack?"

"Hackensack? They still have an Arthur Treacher's Fish and Chips. It's a dump. No. I went straight to 60 Thompson in the Village."

She shot him a knowing look.

"But after dinner I hung out with guys from the music house and we drank PBR at the bar."

"Yeah. Twelve dollar-a-bottle PBR. Any of those guys sporting corn rows or flat-lid trucker caps?"

"Oh shit," Himmelfarb said. "I've become one of them?"

"No, you're becoming one of them. You're trying too hard. Let's just put away the fantasy about drinking rosé wine on the Croisette, and knock this crap out," she said in the calmest demeanor.

She was right. And Himmelfarb never liked not being right.

By the time he got home that night, the kids were sleeping and his wife was in her ratty sweatpants, passed out on the couch. Still stewing over the day's missteps, and dwelling on the missteps of last week, last month, and last year, Himmelfarb plowed through the mail.

A check for $391 from Shelton Square, a limited partnership his father had left him. Though he was knee-deep in the business world, Himmelfarb never understood investments, finance or limited partnerships. But he did enjoy getting unexpected mailbox money.

Of course, the $391 bonus vanished quickly. Bills from the Internet provider, the TV provider and the cell phone provider put him in the hole faster than a planner could deep-six an entire campaign with a simple, "it's not on strategy."

Maybe the strategy isn't on strategy, he so often wanted to fire back at these MBA know-it-alls. How could he be so consistently wrong and everybody else, and their brother, be so consistently right, he asked himself.

The last envelope was from the County of Los Angeles. He recognized it immediately. Himmelfarb was being summoned to Jury Duty. Unlike past summons, on green paper, this one was printed on ominous red paper.

He had failed to appear at the courthouse for three prior occasions and was in danger of violating some obscure Federal ordinance regarding civic responsibility. Could they throw him in jail for not throwing someone else in jail?

Himmelfarb Finds His Mojo

He'd seen enough prison shows to know it wasn't worth the gamble. Besides, he thought, how hard could it be to get out of jury duty?

The Inglewood Courthouse is 10 miles from Himmelfarb's house but it might as well have been 100. Inglewood is a predominantly African American community that has effortlessly avoided gentrification.

The Fabulous Forum, once the home of NBA championships, where Hollywood celebrities would pay $2000 to sit courtside and rub elbows with Magic and Kareem, was now the setting for secondhand flea markets and the occasional raucous Sunday morning Baptist revival.

According to Habeas Corpus, an individual is to be tried fairly before a jury of one's peers. Unless the city of Inglewood had somehow nabbed a cranky, aging, hipster-wannabe ad guy illegally padding his travel expenses, Himmelfarb failed to see how he could be even remotely deemed a peer.

His pasty white skin, made even pastier by the many hours caged in an office seeking the next big idea, stood in contrast to the other African American and Hispanic potential jurors seated in the assembly room.

He struck up a conversation with LaQuisha, a 47-year-old grandmother who lived in the shadow of the Forum for all her days. She'd never been inside the place but always knew when the Lakers were putting on Showtime, just from the roar of the crowds.

"Schvartze?" she asked Himmelfarb.

"It's an old Yiddish term for black people. Not as bad as the N-word, but slightly derogatory. My grandfather used it all the time," Himmelfarb explained, "but that was a long, long time ago."

"And you're gonna tell the judge you don't like schvartzes?" she asked again.

"No. I do like schvartzes. I mean African Americans. We have neighbors in Mar Vista who are African American. They come over for BBQ's all the time. For steak. And sausages. And sometimes chicken...I mean..."

"I know what you mean."

"I don't have time for jury duty. I have to get back to work. We're launching Snugget, a new candy bar. Frap Jacks, squeezable pancake batter in a tube. And we're pitching Tomsk, the first Russian automobile in the United States."

"That's important stuff. I can see why you'd want to play the race card," said LaQuisha.

"You don't think it's a good idea?"

"Oh, that might get you out of jury duty but you may have a harder time getting out of Inglewood."

She picked up her iPhone, as if to dismiss any further conversation, and resumed her online game of Candy Crush. Moments later, the bailiff called for Juror #492, LaQuisha.

"You say you would be unable to render a fair judgment if called to serve, could you elaborate on that?" asked the District Attorney.

She paused, took a deep breath, and gave herself a moment to spot Himmelfarb in the crowd.

"First of all, let me say, I have nothing against white people, I like white folk. I just don't know if I can trust them."

"So," the District Attorney followed, "if I were to present evidence to you indicating the guilt of the defendant, you would question the truth of that evidence simply because I am a white man?"

Himmelfarb Finds His Mojo

"I know it sounds stupid and irrational but yes. Yes, I would."

"The District Attorney's office asks that this juror be excused."

LaQuisha bounced from her seat and bolted for the double doors at the rear of the courtroom. As she passed Himmelfarb she made it a point to stop, place a warm hand over his and whisper, "Good luck, honey. I'm sure this roomful of schvartzes can't wait until you take the stand."

She was followed by a cavalcade of prospective jurors, each more inventive and more determined than the previous to have themselves excused from service.

There was Juror #265, the outspoken Latina with the bad acne.

She had a huge chip on her shoulder and wanted the world, or at least Inglewood, to know she planned on making something of herself. Before the District Attorney fired off the first question, she had pre-emptively rattled off her entire resume.

Not only had this woman graduated from Long Beach Community College, she was going to be taking the LSATs and getting into law school.

Every question was answered with another question. Or worse, a rambling cyclical time-consuming rant that was intended to demonstrate her verbal prowess but instead made her the most hated person in the room – a room housing two alleged rapists, three car thieves and a nun charged with embezzling funds from an orphanage.

"Dismissed."

She was followed by Juror #359, the other male Caucasian summoned to Inglewood that day.

Himmelfarb Finds His Mojo

Earlier, Himmelfarb stood behind him at the corner Starbucks, where in perfect English, he nonchalantly ordered a Double Shot Venti Americano with extra whip and a pinch of cinnamon. But somewhere between the coffee stand and the panel box, the man had affected a near-perfect Russian accent as well as a convincing inability to understand the simplest English instruction.

"What you mean, take oath?"

"Dismissed."

When the proceedings weren't comical, they were downright pathetic.

Juror #421 told a riveting tale about how her parents had been murdered in a home invasion robbery. Her brother shot down on the streets of Gardena. And her sister incarcerated for trafficking drugs, carjacking and threatening a neighbor with a machete.

"Dismissed."

She giggled as she skipped out of the courtroom, leaving the already shallow jury pool that much shallower.

Himmelfarb, an advertising man who had always pictured himself atop the Bullshitter's Food Chain, was clearly out of his league. By the time his number was called, all the good excuses, all the dramatics, all the possible reasons for not having to sit in the box had been taken.

He answered every question with an efficient, monosyllabic yes or no. Both sides must have felt like they had hit the jury jackpot.

To the District Attorney, Himmelfarb was a property-owning, gainfully employed father of twins with a stake in keeping our streets peaceful and orderly.

Himmelfarb Finds His Mojo

To the defense team, he was a college-educated Westsider with an abiding sense of fairness and a full-sized SUV packed to the gills with white guilt.

"Accepted."

"Accepted."

And there it was. Himmelfarb, already four days into the slog through our nation's judicial system, was now looking at considerably more time.

What would he draw? A burglary? A hit-and-run? What if he landed on some murder case and had to spend the next six months of his life in sequestration, quarantined off from the world at the Inglewood Comfort Inn, with dial-up Internet and black and white TV? Who would introduce America to the newest confectionary sensation, Snugget?

The best he could hope for was an open and shut case.

"Good morning," said the D.A., "I want to thank you all for agreeing to serve on the jury. It is an honor to have you here. Now if I could ask you all to take a look at this videotape."

Videotape? What about the eloquent opening statement? The passionate plea for justice? The classic Clarence Darrow Gambit?

This was like a third string quarterback throwing a 70-yard Hail Mary pass on the first play from scrimmage. And scoring.

The bailiff lowered the lights and the jury turned its attention to the large screen set up next to the judge's bench.

From a security camera mounted on the ceiling, they saw a small elderly Pakistani man behind the counter of a 7-11. As he counted the batteries stocked on the display rack and marked the inventory down on a clipboard, a tall, bespectacled African-American man wearing a golf shirt, navy blue shorts and distinctive tennis shoes entered the store. In his right hand, and in clear view of the HD camera, was a foot-long flathead screwdriver.

Within seconds, he was behind the counter and towering over the Pakistani, who hadn't been in the country long enough to recognize any suspicious behavior. But it didn't take long for Roger (perhaps the Americanized version of Raja or just a name the Pakistani liked) to realize he was being robbed. With the screwdriver pressed into his back and in strict compliance with the 7-11 training manual, Roger offered no resistance. He quickly emptied both cash registers and handed over the bounty, all of $54.

The thief ran out the door and Roger immediately dialed 911.

"Yes...yes...I just have been robbed....Very, big black man. Very black...yes...yes. 7-11...down the street...on La Brea...right next to police station...very big black man..." said Roger, gasping to take a breath.

"He took all the money...no, I am not hurt...can you hold on one second?"

Roger placed the receiver of the phone on the counter. The videotape showed a customer, who had been at the back of the store and missed the robbery, placing some merchandise in front of Roger, a man with an unstoppable work ethic.

"Ok, raspberry ice tea and BBQ Doritos, anything else sir? $4.83. Do you have a five? I am just now all out of singles. Thank you very much. Have a nice night."

Roger picked up the phone and without missing a beat, "Send the police here, right away...yes, I have been robbed."

Himmelfarb Finds His Mojo

Taking a time out in the middle of a 911 emergency call to ring up an ice tea and some chemically-flavored chips was probably not in the 7-11 training manual, but it did bring howling laughter to the entire courtroom and made Roger feel like a minor celebrity. The old man was smiling from one edge of his turban to the other.

Himmelfarb thought he had won the lottery. A textbook late night robbery, all captured on videotape, all in stunning High Definition clarity. It doesn't get any more open and shut than this.

The defense attorney thought otherwise.

If the junior lawyer from prestigious Southwestern University could swing an acquittal here, anything was possible. He could get out of public defending. He could land a job at some swanky law firm in Hawthorne. And get his hands on that shiny new Chevy Malibu he'd been eyeing, the one with the power door locks and power mirrors.

This could be the beginning, the aspiring defense attorney thought. All it took was some 'reasonable doubt.' Reasonable doubt, however, was not going to be easy in this case.

Shortly after the robbery and moments after Roger called in to the authorities, the police apprehended a tall African American man wearing the same beige golf shirt, navy blue shorts and distinctive tennis shoes as the man at the 7-11. Moreover, in his pocket they found a large flathead screwdriver and $54, the exact amount stolen from the convenience store.

Two officers took the stand and identified the man sitting at the defense table as the same man in the videotape. Although, and this was the defense attorney's shining opportunity, the man apprehended, after a quarter mile foot chase through the backstreets of Inglewood, was *not* wearing glasses.

The burglar on the videotape *was* wearing glasses.

Himmelfarb Finds His Mojo

The lawyer's "AHA!" moment was short-circuited by the fleet-footed patrolman who said the glasses fell off in the scuffle. In fact, an hour after he was booked, the police retraced the route of the foot chase and found the glasses in question.

Undeterred, or perhaps just clutching at straws, the defense attorney gamely posited that at some point in our lives we have all approached someone walking on the street and greeted them with a hello, a hug or a handshake. Only to recognize, split seconds later, that the person is a doppelganger for a friend or family member.

"Isn't is possible," he asked, "that this is simply a case of mistaken identity?"

The defense rested.

The bailiff guided Himmelfarb and his 11 fellow jurists into a small chamber room behind the judge's bench. Instead of a long stately table, as seen in *12 Angry Men*, there was a large circular table that looked like it had been rolled out of a Chinatown restaurant. All it lacked was soy sauce and a Lazy Susan.

"Please pass the verdicts and the Kung Pao Chicken."

The bailiff left them with a few simple instructions.

"Pick a jury foreman and when you've reached a unanimous decision ring this bell."

The seats were still cold when the Juror #167, an Asian woman in her mid-fifties turned to Himmelfarb and nominated him for foremen.

"Why me?" he said reflexively.

"You, you smart man," replied the woman.

"No. Not smart," Himmelfarb protested, not wanting the responsibility.

"You smart. You show up every day on time. You speak good English. You smart. And you no watch Jerry Springer on waiting room television," she stated.

There was a good deal of head nodding. Reluctantly, Himmelfarb accepted the position and did what any newbie Jury Foreman would do, he called for a vote. He folded and ripped a blank piece of paper and distributed the little scraplets to the eleven strangers who would decide the defendant's fate. Each grabbed a pencil from the middle of the table where the soy sauce and stewed hot peppers would have been.

"Guilty."
"Guilty."
"Guilty."
"Guilty."
"Guilty."
"Guilty."
"Guilty."
"Guilty."
"Guilty."
"Guilty."
"Guilty."

"Undecided."

"What?" exclaimed Pat, the woman to Himmelfarb's immediate left, a feisty 62 year old, who wanted nothing more than to get out of this courthouse and back to her soap operas.

Then, addressing the man who scribbled Undecided, "Do I have to come around this table and smack the silly out of you?"

Himmelfarb Finds His Mojo

Himmelfarb liked Pat. They sat next to each other in the jury box and she always seemed to enjoy his little snarky asides.

When the day's proceedings were concluded, he would often walk Pat back to her car, a '72 pitch black Buick Electra 225 that was her late husband's pride and joy. While Himmelfarb coveted the 'Deuce and a Quarter', he also enjoyed her colorful stories about early Inglewood, before its decline.

When it came time to take this doubting Thomas out to the woodshed, Pat was more than up to the task.

"What do you mean undecided?" she barked.

"I mean I'm undecided. What if the man the police caught is not the same man on the videotape? There could have been 100 guys walking through Inglewood at 2 in the morning with a flat head screwdriver and $54 in their pocket," said the lone holdout. "And the man in the courtroom was not wearing glasses."

"Boy, I have seen stupid in my day, but you are the Marion Barry of stupid," said Pat.

She was just winding up.

"I wear glasses. And when I go to bed or I take a shower or my late dear husband Freddy made sweet love to me, I do not wear glasses. If my lawyer said the only way to keep me out of a San Quentin jail cell was to not wear glasses, I would take those glasses and grind them up in the garbage disposal. Now get out those pieces of paper and let's take another vote because Ruby is about to dump Tony and run away with her lesbian lover Elena and I am not about to miss my soaps because of some dumbass fool who never heard of contact lenses. Undecided! My ass, in two parts."

They voted again. This time there was no dissent.

Ten minutes later the cuffs were slapped on the defendant and he was whisked away to exchange his thrift store bought blazer and slacks for an orange jumpsuit, provided by the Department of Corrections and the good people of California.

All for $54.

Himmelfarb walked Pat back to her Buick. He couldn't shake a nagging thought.

"Why do you suppose he went to all the trouble? There was videotape, the cops caught him red-handed right after the robbery, it was a slam-dunk. So why not plead it out an maybe get a lighter sentence?" he asked.

"Are you serious, honey?" Pat replied.

"I guess I am," said Himmelfarb who was genuinely confused.

"Child, that man was guilty. Everybody knows he was guilty. You. Me. Raja. The defense lawyer. He was a two-striker."

"A two-striker?"

"He had two prior convictions. If he pleads guilty to a third, he gets sent away for life. So he took his chances. Thinking some witless clown might let him off the hook. Losers like that are why the Lakers left Inglewood."

"And the Kings."

"Oh who gives a damn about hockey?"

Himmelfarb was stunned by her street smarts. That little nugget of wisdom never occurred to him.

Himmelfarb Finds His Mojo

He realized then that he probably would never see Pat or the Electra or even Inglewood ever again. And that his whole jury duty experience was not altogether unpleasant.

For a week and a half he enjoyed the company of people who had never heard of JWT or DDB or TBWA. People who didn't speak of content creation. Or going viral. Or 720 degrees of fully scalable data-driven integration.

People who didn't give a damn about advertising and saw it for what it was, noxious emissions from the engine of capitalism.

"Hey, you want to go out for lunch? I'm buying," said Himmelfarb.

Pat turned to him, "Darling, if you're buying, I'm dining."

"What about your soap operas?"

"It's all going on the DVR."

They got in the Buick and shut the massive heavy doors.

Pat added, "Don't you white people know anything?"

Feldman Goes Deaf

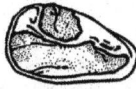

prime rib

Feldman Goes Deaf

"I'm sorry, I didn't hear you," asked a very puzzled Dr. Greenblatt. "Did you say you wanted me to sever your eardrums?"

Feldman replied, "That's exactly what I said."

The doctor, who had been administering medicine for more than 35 years, closed the door to his Midtown office. He knew what troubled Feldman, could not be fixed with a scalpel. He settled into his creaky leather chair and using nothing more than body language, invited his new patient to explain.

"...It's everything Doc, from barking dogs to colicky babies. It's nonstop. It all comes in, but it has no place to go. I just want some silence. I want to be alone with my thoughts."

"I understand," said the doctor.

"For God's sake, I don't need to be alerted every time a truck driver puts his vehicle in reverse..."

Feldman was shifting from first gear into second.

"I read this article the other day. It said, *How to Get Ahead in Business by Being a Better Listener*. It was all about collaboration. About taking constructive criticism. And building consensus with the team."

The doctor edged in a word, "Was it helpful?"

"If it was helpful, I wouldn't be in your office requesting the Helen Keller surgery," steamed Feldman, who now had it third gear.

Feldman Goes Deaf

"I have no interest in building consensus with the team. I don't even want to be on a team. I don't want to collaborate with anybody. I'm not interested in feedback. Less input, more output. That's what I say."

Dr. Greenblatt checked his charts. "You're a playwright, is that correct?"

Feldman corrected him, "I *was* a playwright. Nobody goes to live theater anymore."

He glared at Dr. Greenblatt.

"When was the last time you took your wife to the theater?"

Suddenly on the defensive, the doctor offered," Well, we get Netflix. And my wife has..."

"Damn Netflix," Feldman interrupted.

At which point the doctor decided it wasn't worth telling him of his wife's rheumatoid arthritis and how it left her homebound.

"The whole world comes streaming into your home. Why would anybody go see actors on stage acting, when with the click of a mouse they can stream a movie? Or worse, some crap on YouTube. You know what killed live theater in New York City? Cat videos. God-damned cat videos."

The doctor snuck a glance at Feldman's chart to see if his blood pressure was elevated.

It was.

"For the last two years I've been writing infomercials. Portable grills, electric pet hairbrushes and magical brass polishers. The money is good. It pays the bills. Keeps the ex-wife happy in her little Chelsea townhouse. And happy ex-wife equals happy life."

At least this crazy former playwright has medical insurance, the doctor thought to himself.

"But I have to sit in meetings and listen to the most dimwitted cretins on the planet. We spent all of last week debating whether the call to action should say 'learn more' or 'discover more'. Pie charts. Data analytics. A 1,400 page Powerpoint. A whole fucking week. I've never seen so many people accomplishing so little."

Feldman was now in fourth gear.

The doctor said, "We all have to put up with the indignities of life. I'm not sure how yours merit such an odd and extreme surgical solution?"

"The other day, I'm in my office and the phone rings. There was a time when I had a creative assistant who would screen my calls so I could focus my attention on writing the infomercials, you know the stuff that keeps the electricity going for the company."

Greenblatt pushed his seat back ever so slightly.

"But I don't have an office anymore. I sit at a big picnic table. In what they call an open office plan. I don't have a creative assistant anymore. I don't have anyone anymore. I do have 20 other people. Sitting on my left. And my right. I don't know what they do. Half the time they're playing with their iWatches or their FitJits. So now I have to answer the phone. And who is it?"

The doctor had no idea who it was.

"Cal Sweetbaum, the client. Cal the Copywriter, he calls himself. No one else calls him that. Cal thinks he has a way with words. He has a way with turds."

Adding, "Three weeks ago I hand in a 45 page draft for some new waffle maker. Some *farkakte* device that cooks waffles in half the time.

"Let me ask you something, Doc? When was the last time you ate a waffle?"

"...errrr..."

"Exactly. People don't eat waffles. OK, some do. But research shows people who eat waffles, do so once every three months. So if you're waiting three months for your next waffle, how important is it to shave that time down by four minutes?"

The doctor was trying to track Feldman, who was now clearly riding the red line.

"But what do I know? I wrote the damn script. Not one of my best, but not one of my worst either. Then I hand it in to Cal the Copywriter."

The doctor could tell this wasn't going to end well.

"Then Cal – I don't even like the sound of his name – tells me he has some other direction he'd like me to explore," said Feldman, "How many goddamned directions can there be to selling a waffle maker?"

"So now I have to start from scratch and spend the next two and half weeks doing it the way Cal would have written it, you know, if Cal had any ability to write it in the first place."

Feldman sat back in his seat. He took a deep breath to calm himself and added, "I can't take it anymore, Doctor. I need a way to turn it all off. Can you help me?"

"I can help you," replied the doctor.

"Excellent," said Feldman, letting out the last bit of carbon dioxide left in his lungs.

"But not in the way you're asking."

Dr. Greenblatt stood up from his chair, walked over to the bookcase and retrieved a small *masu*, a wooden box used to drink sake during Japanese ceremonies. It was painted with a deep, black lacquer. There was stack of rice paper business cards inside the box. He handed one to Feldman.

He had never seen a business card like this before. On the front of was a small blue circle. It was embossed on the card in thick, shiny ink, and rose up like half an M&M. On the back, in the tiniest of type, was a Park Ave. address. Feldman marveled at the simple beauty of this business card. It had an aesthetic unlike anything he'd ever seen.

"Go see Dennis."

Feldman ran his thumb over the blue dot as he walked the eight blocks back to his office. As he waited on the corner of 47th and Madison, Feldman scanned the mass of humanity going about their noisy midtown business.

He spotted a young man carrying a leather portfolio, perhaps a budding photographer or architect. The young man seemed lost. Feldman watched and eavesdropped as the young artist approached an older gentlemen standing next to a hot dog cart.

"Excuse me sir, do you know how I can get to this address?" the young man showed him a scratch of paper.

"Yes. You go two blocks west and make a right at 5th Ave.," the New Yorker respectfully obliged. "It'll be right there."

"Are you sure?" the younger man mistakenly inquired again.

Feldman Goes Deaf

"You asked me. I told you," the old-time New Yorker snapped, "What am I, Rand 'Fuckin' McNally?"

The sudden ugliness of the old man's voice made Feldman cringe. He pressed harder on the blue dot.

On Monday, he found himself in the lobby of the Park Ave. co-op. He scanned the building directory. There, between the Murphy's, the Cohen's and Magliano's, he spotted a single blue dot. No name. Just a graphic blue dot.

Without the exchange of a single word, he was buzzed in. He rode alone in the silent elevator and stood nervously before the door of apartment 1001.

"I am Dennis. Please come in."

Dennis was hardly the imposing Zen Master that Feldman had imagined. He had no long white flowing beard. His eyes were almond-shaped. And he came to the door in cargo shorts and a Tommy Bahama silk shirt. He looked more like a Hawaiian tourist than a fount of ancient Eastern mystical secrets. If not for the unmistakable smell of incense and the new age sound of Smooth Jazz, Feldman might have done an about-face and headed back to Dr. Greenblatt's.

He entered the cavernous apartment, the sound of his footsteps swallowed by the thickest carpet he'd ever set foot on. He was immediately disoriented by the height of the ceilings. They were 30 feet high.

"I bought the apartment above mine and then I gutted it to increase my cubic space and give the place a more airy feel," Dennis explained.

"That must have cost a fortune. And you didn't increase your square footage by one inch. That's not very smart." Feldman said, his filter turned completely off.

"Space is its own reward," replied Dennis.

"OK, this guy is a major loon," Feldman thought to himself. On the other hand, it was this bit of remodeling irrationality that gave Dennis Kim instant credibility.

"I spoke with Dr. Greenblatt about your request and he has filled me in on your personal history. So we can proceed right away."

One last hurdle stood before Feldman and the promise of blessed peace and quiet. They took a seat at Mr. Kim's 400 year old, hand-carved teak desk to hammer out the financials.

"I'm almost afraid to ask..." he stumbled.

Mr. Kim interrupted, "I know. You are wondering about the cost."

"Well, I know it's not covered by my insurance."

"No, this is elective, so it is not," said Mr. Kim. "But you need not worry. I think you'll find the price very reasonable." He picked up a calligraphy pen to write on a small piece of paper. He folded it in two and passed it across the desk.

Feldman steeled himself before looking at the paper. What could 'reasonable' mean to a man who owned 400 year old furniture and who had committed virtual real estate suicide?

"Before you look at the cost I want you to realize that I cannot take away your hearing in one fell swoop. It will require some time and a regimen."

Fair enough, thought Feldman, who gingerly opened the folded up piece of paper.

"This is the price per session, right?" he asked.

Feldman Goes Deaf

"Oh, no," said Dennis. "That covers the entire program."

Feldman was shocked. Pleasantly shocked. He couldn't square away Mr. Kim's fee with Mr. Kim's opulent surroundings. Perhaps he's a volume guy, thought Feldman.

The following week he began the program designed to render him completely deaf.

Dennis explained how the eardrums were no different than any other organ in the body. They could be trained. Mastered. Turned on and off.

He seated Feldman in a plain wooden chair. Then he rolled out an ancient gong recovered from the castle of a 6th century *shogun* warlord. The first gong hits were the worst. Every time, Feldman flinched or reacted to the loud sound, he would receive the quick micro-snap of a bamboo cane to the most sensitive point on his chin.

Gong.
Snap.
Gong.
Snap.
Gong.
Snap.

The pain was excruciating. But Feldman, having grown up watching David Carradine in the TV show *Kung Fu*, convinced himself that if Shaolin monks could walk on broken glass and lift scolding urns with their forearms, he could endure this temporary sting to turn off a world of non-stop noise.

When he had successfully remained still in the face of a banging gong, Mr. Kim had him turn his seat around so he could no longer associate the sound with the sight.

Feldman Goes Deaf

Each week was followed by a new technique.

There were hot Bikram Yoga sessions, performed in a sweating room where the temperature never dipped below 100. Long periods of silent meditation. And an endless supply of a foul tasting concoction of lemon juice, cayenne peppers and vanilla extract that Mr. Kim promised would hasten the results.

Once, while silently reading in unison with Mr. Kim from an old book of Chinese poetry, Feldman looked up and noticed a wall of framed 8x10 glossy photos. These were not celebrities of the *People* Magazine variety. These were CEO's, politicians, Nobel Prize winners, men and women who had, through the force of their will, advanced civilization.

"All former clients," beamed Mr. Kim.

Feldman blurted, "That's Steve..."

"That's right," interrupted Dennis. "He came to me years ago. Said he wanted to turn the computer industry on its head. He wanted to change everything. From the way we listen to music to the way we watch video."

"He came to you?"

"Sat right where you're sitting. You can't make those kind of seismic shifts when you're constantly distracted. You have to be focused. You have to tune out all the doubt and all those who would have you compromise," said Dennis. "When the mind is free..."

Kim looked up and caught Feldman staring at him.

Feldman could see that Kim's mouth was moving, but nothing seemed to be coming out. He leaned forward. Nothing.

Feldman Goes Deaf

Mr. Kim went to his desk and retrieved a boating air horn. Everyone in the apartment building heard it. Feldman did not.

He was now officially deaf.

He strolled through midtown Manhattan as if it were the first time he'd ever seen the place. It smelled different.

He saw cabbies weaving in and out of traffic, coming within a hair's breadth of each other. He knew they were honking their horns. But he didn't hear it.

He didn't hear the sleazy sidewalk merchants hawking their imitation luxury luggage.

He didn't hear the Persian dealmakers barking their demands into their Bluetooth headsets.

He didn't hear the bearded homeless vets begging for whiskey change.

It was all blissfully gone. New York felt new again.

Back at the office, Feldman smiled at the receptionist, whose voice had always grated on him.

"Morning, Mr. Feldman," she said in her singsong voice.

He, of course, could not hear her, but saw her sickening saccharine smile and returned her greeting with a grin, a wink and a surreal cheeriness that no one would ever associate with Feldman.

Later that morning he went to the mandatory status meeting.

Here, the young coordinators and ambitious project managers would wield their power and talk about the projects others would have to start working on. No detail or looming deadline was too insignificant. And though all the vitals were clearly spelled out on paper or in a stream of endless emails that would follow the meeting, they somehow needed to be vocalized.

Over and over and over again.

Feldman hated status meetings. He dreaded them more than the ride home on the number 7 line. Where he would often find himself wedged between loud, arguing Filipino families, or surrounded by high school kids who took the phrase 'finger-licking good chicken' way too literally.

But today was a new day. And the status meeting was not the status quo.

While the minions took on the minutia of the day, Feldman played online chess on his smartphone and took on random newcomers. He joyously delivered a knockout knight/rook/pawn combination to Heinz3489, who hailed from Hamburg. To reward himself, he sauntered over to the snack tray and indulged in a blueberry bear claw, which he had always resisted in the past.

His newfound deafness was paying huge dividends.

Whereas before he found himself accommodating his coworkers' deficiencies and their slovenly work ethic, now the tables had been turned. They had to adapt to his sudden unexplainable loss of hearing.

There was a 2:00 P.M. conference call. Cal the Copywriter wanted to go over his latest revisions on the WaffleTron 9000. Feldman gladly accepted the meeting invite and was the first to show up.

Not wanting to open up a can of worms, the account people prefaced the meeting with a little white lie about Feldman's laryngitis. They took copious notes as Cal detailed his wish for a more thorough romancing of the patented non-stick Teflon surface.

Feldman Goes Deaf

The Cal conference call lasted more than an hour. Feldman hadn't checked his watch once.

They reviewed footage of waffle batter pouring onto a griddle. And got into a heated discussion about the merits of take #17 versus take #31. One had a near perfect smooth flow, while the other had tantalizing batter bubbles that potential waffle-making machine buyers would find irresistible.

Feldman didn't hear a word of the insanity. Nor did he care.

He returned to his numerous games of online chess and pounded a stockbroker from Chicago with a brutal queen/knight attack. He dispatched a newbie from New Mexico. And he found a worthy adversary from Finland who thoroughly tested his endgame skills.

Later that day, an account executive showed up in his office. She had transcribed the entire meeting. More importantly, the account team had done what they had never done before. They prepared a topline report. Condensing all the vital points of the meeting into a concise one-page report. They even took the time to draw up an action plan so that the entire WaffleTron 9000 team would know how to proceed in exact accordance with the client's wishes.

In essence they rendered Feldman's attendance of the meeting completely unnecessary. A point he had made countless times before but had somehow fallen on deaf ears.

Radio silence suited Feldman.

Co-workers found him more agreeable. Less given to ranting, mostly because he had little to rant about.

Had you asked, even fellow strap-hangers on the number 7 Line would tell you how much nicer it was not to be on the receiving end of Feldman's ugly scowls.

Feldman Goes Deaf

He even re-upped the lease on his outrageously expensive apartment. And he despised living in that apartment, 22B. Feldman swore his landlord harbored a personal vendetta against him and went out of his way to rent out 23B, the apartment above him, to drummers. Tap dancers. And drummers who dabbled in tap dancing.

None of that mattered anymore.

Let others seek the Fountain of Youth. The secret to happiness, according to Feldman, was finding life's great big Mute Button.

His birthday arrived and though he had no plans for a party or even a lunch with co-workers, it was going to be Feldman's best birthday ever.

After many revisions and tweaks between the agency and America's foremost manufacturer of waffle making machines, the infomercial had been shot, edited and shipped for air. His longstanding national waffle-making nightmare was over.

Because of his newfound agreeability, Feldman earned himself a raise and an office. A real office. With a door. A door that could be opened, and more importantly, closed.

Feldman, with his acutely working four senses all dialed up to 11, had it all. If life could be better, he couldn't imagine how.

Before his subway ride home, he stopped in at Pakula's Deli. It wasn't a big deli and never had the cachet of Katz's or Second Ave. But to those who knew pastrami, and Feldman knew pastrami, Pakula's was the only game in town.

Because it was his birthday, he ordered the full sandwich. On toasted crisp rye. With a light smattering of spicy brown mustard and a thin layer of tangy sauerkraut.

Feldman Goes Deaf

It smelled so good, he was tempted to rip open the bag and eat it right there from the comfort of his graffiti-marked plastic subway seat.

But he knew better. And the perfect complement to this culinary masterpiece, a frosty 24-ounce Tsingtao beer, was just minutes away in his refrigerator.

He eased into his leather recliner and set the glorious feast before him on the coffee table. He turned on the television and cued up a previously recorded episode of *Jeopardy*, close-captioned for Feldman's enjoyment. Just as he was set to take that long anticipated first bite of Pakula's fabulously unfamous pastrami, his smartphone began to vibrate. He looked at the screen and his face fell.

It was his daughter, calling from Australia. He hadn't spoken to her for a while. She called to wish him a happy birthday. But it was no regular call. She had used the FaceTime feature on her phone because she had a special gift.

Her son, Jeremy, Feldman's grandson, was now 18 months old. He was walking. And talking. And singing.

Happy Birthday to you.
Happy Birthday to you.
Happy Birthday, dear Papa.
Happy Birthday to you.

Feldman never heard a word of it.

He grabbed the small whiteboard he had been using to communicate with the plumber, electrician and the pizza delivery boy. He scratched out a note to his daughter, and grandson, that he lost his voice and asked if she could call back later.

"OK, later Papa. We love you."

Feldman Goes Deaf

Feldman hung up the phone and stared at his sandwich. He never took a bite of it. The pastrami sandwich stared back at him the very next morning, the day after his not-so-happy birthday.

Feldman dashed off an email to his office. He wasn't coming in that day. He spent the rest of the morning tearing through his apartment until he found the unusual rice paper business card with the blue dot.

He returned to the Park Ave. co-op owned by Master Kim, who was not at all surprised to see him. He invited him to the unexplainably large apartment and had him take a seat on the new custom-made Italian sofa.

"I want my hearing back."

Dennis smiled.

"Can you reverse the process?"

Dennis smiled again. And nodded.

"How much will it cost?"

Dennis held up a finger as if to say, "Wait here." He slowly walked over to his desk to retrieve his calligraphy pen and a small piece of paper. He came back into the living room and wrote a number on the paper. He folded the paper in two and slid it across the table to Feldman.

Feldman opened the folded piece of paper and, like before, he was shocked.

Unlike the last time, this time it was not so pleasant.

The Coach Who Would Not Speak

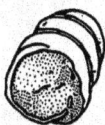

rolled roast

The Coach Who Would Not Speak

The Southern California Chrysler Plymouth Dealers hated Pat Riley.

Hated him.

This, despite the fact that Riley coached Magic Johnson, Kareem Abdul Jabbar, and James Worthy, to five World Championships. To the dealers, that meant nothing. Pat Riley was no better than the appropriately named Red Klotz, the owner/coach of the Washington Generals, who battled bravely but never beat their archrivals, the Harlem Globetrotters.

They weren't always sour on Pat. For years he was their guy. They had him make celebrity appearances at dealer functions. Give motivational speeches. And shill their cars, quite successfully, on locally run TV commercials.

But that all changed in 1992 on a Chrysler Plymouth Dealership floor in Van Nuys, California.

And Glen Tochterman was there to witness it all.

Perhaps it was the end-of-the-year doldrums, or the sagging economy, but for some mysterious reason, which had nothing to do with shoddy craftsmanship, piss-poor gas mileage and Ukrainian-inspired ergonomics, people were not scooping up the newest offerings from Chrysler Plymouth.

The yacht-like Imperials were gathering dust. No one was loving the lavish New Yorker. And the boxy Horizon was clearly a decade ahead of its time.

Later, those unsightly angular lines and Bauhausian look would be a big hit when they reappeared in the Pontiac Aztec. But for now, and for the lowly Horizon, it was a No Sale.

Glen knew that when the dealers aren't selling cars and the factory isn't making any worth selling, the problem ends up in the sorry lap of the advertising agency.

That can only mean one thing: A Tent Sale. Because as copywriter Glen Tochterman would often say, "Sales rise when you merchandise."

A Tent Sale is a lot like the Creationist theory. There's no evidence or hard data to support it. No one has ever produced any meaningful research on its efficacy. But just as people will flock to a tent revival on a Sunday morning for spiritual nourishment, they also believe they can get a better deal on a car when it is displayed under a large canopy with broad red and white stripes

Praise the Lord.

Perhaps it stems from that old maxim coined by legendary Studebaker salesman Tom Parker, who in 1953 at a dealership outside Peoria, famously said, "The tent is going up, and the prices are going down."

The first part of the shoot had gone extremely well. Riley's hair had been greased back to perfection. His crisp Armani suit looked stunning. And his delivery was flawless. He power-walked through the maze of shiny new cars, hit all his marks and gave Tochterman's amateurish copy just the right amount of smile and energy.

"You'll be driving the lane in style in this luxurious new New Yorker."

"This Acclaim is a slam dunk."

"You drive home in this K car, and I get the assist."

The Coach Who Would Not Speak

With any luck, Tochterman thought, this 14-hour shoot should be wrapped up in 12. But Glen Tochterman didn't have any luck that day, least of all good luck.

At the last minute, Frank Tompkins, a dealer from San Diego who was fond of polyester suits and big boobed strippers, requested a change on the scripts. Frank wanted Coach Riley to slap the hood of a maroon Le Baron and announce there was a $2000 factory cash back incentive.

Frank thought it was good idea, Riley did not. He blew the whistle and called a personal foul.

The shooting screeched to a grinding halt. And Coach made it abundantly clear that he was not about to read any lines that had to do with cash incentives, discounts or rebates. Or frankly, anything that sprung from the mouth of Frank Tompkins.

It was below him and not in keeping with the celebrity brand he had worked so hard to establish.

Tochterman face-palmed himself.

Damn, he thought, a shill is a shill is a shill. We, Riles, the dealers, the ad agency executives, the electricians, the key grips, the caterers, the guy who brings around those mystery-meat-wrapped-in-lettuce-cup things, we're all on the set that day for one purpose: to sell more Chryslers. To Tochterman, it appeared the Coach was not being a good team player. What difference does it make if he says $2000 cash back?

On the other hand, he reasoned, Coach had a reputation to protect and a future to consider. A future that hopefully did not include any more lowbrow, sheet metal-pounding commercials for local car dealer associations.

The Coach Who Would Not Speak

Like any good actor throwing a tantrum on the set, Coach Riley announced, "I'll be in my trailer."

And with that he was off to his luxuriously appointed, mini-Airstream parked in the back of the dealer lot, behind a fleet of mothballed Horizons.

Pat was not budging. And the dealers were not budging. That put the onus on Glen Tochterman, a junior writer who was only shooting his seventh TV commercial.

For the next five hours Tochterman scrambled to rewrite scripts that would soothe both parties. It felt like another Camp David Summit, only in this case the parties were more entrenched than the Arabs or the Israelis.

Compromises were made. Sloppy graphics were drawn up. And more bad basketball puns were tossed in the air. A day that began with so much promise ended 19 hours later. No one left the set happy.

A week later, Coach Pat Riley was released from his contract with the Southern California Chrysler Plymouth Dealers.

That might have been a great learning experience for some businesses, but advertising isn't like other businesses. Advertising people don't learn from mistakes. They keep repeating them.

Politicians double down.
Ad people double double down.

So instead of embarking on a new, fresher direction that didn't require a celebrity spokesperson, the dealers and the agency brass, agreed to get a new celebrity spokesperson. Someone instantly recognizable. A member with good standing in the Chrysler Plymouth family. A celebrity who could do the dealership power walk and was willing to say all the things Coach Riley wouldn't.

The Coach Who Would Not Speak

Fade in on Ricardo Montalban.

The choice actually made sense, since years earlier Mr. Montalban appeared in a national commercial for the Chrysler Cordoba, with its signature, "Rich Corinthian Leather." For a short while those three marketing-manufactured words enjoyed catchphrase status and were repeated by stand up comedians and dropped into parody skits on Saturday Night Live.

The truth is there's no such thing. The leather in Chryslers doesn't come from Corinthia. It comes from Newark, NJ – widely agreed to be the birthplace of the first carjacking.

Glen Tochterman looked forward to meeting Mr. Montalban, who chose not to come into the agency for the meaningless tour of the cubicle farm and instead opted for a casual sit down lunch at a snazzy restaurant in Brentwood.

Ricardo was not a fan of large groups and preferred to keep things more intimate. There, he made instant friends with Glen Tochterman and Julia the broadcast producer on the project.

He took an immediate liking to Julia, though she was a good 30 years younger. Perhaps even mistaking her for a Latina, due in large part to her dark Slavic complexion. In subsequent meetings he'd always request Julia to be present. And was never shy about his feelings towards her.

"Ahhhh, Julia, so glad you could make it. You are so very attrrrrrractive."

Naturally, he rolled the "r's", giving the pronunciation its own distinctive flair. And amply demonstrating why non-existent Rich Corinthian Leather lives in the minds of millions.

Knowing of the problems with Coach Riley and perhaps fancying the opportunity to bring about a late resurgence in his career, Mr.

The Coach Who Would Not Speak

Montalban was keen on having weekly meetings to monitor the progress of the new campaign. He also made it a point to generously spread the flattery.

Julia might have been very attractive, but Mr. Montalban was equally smitten with Glen Tochterman, who he claimed had a fertile imagination. As the camaraderie grew, so did the pile of approved scripts Mr. Montalban agreed to film.

After weeks of creative development, tweaking and re-tweaking, Tochterman had three fully fleshed out campaigns. And as Mr. Montalban, a veteran of countless feature films and TV shows, put it, "I'd be happy to appear in any of the work they choose."

Naturally, Tochterman's confidence soared. It isn't everyday that a legitimate Hollywood actor says something as heartening as, "I wouldn't change a word."

They were almost at the finish line.

The team assembled at the posh Los Angeles Athletic Club to present the new campaigns to 25 of the most powerful Chrysler Plymouth dealers. These included the local salesman but also some out of town delegates from other regions who were thinking about jumping on board the Ricardo Montalban bandwagon.

Furthermore, Bozell Advertising, the agency of record, decided to send some heavyweights from the NY office to make sure the client was happy. And stayed happy.

There was enough pressure in that room for three presentations.

After a series of charts and slides offered up by the account people and the planners, it was Tochterman's turn to put on the dog and pony and Montalban show.

The Coach Who Would Not Speak

It was, in his mind, the perfect presentation. Tochterman paced out the setups. He eased through the copy with nary a stumble. And then, when the timing couldn't have been any better, he delivered the carefully crafted, Montalban-approved punch lines with the seasoned flair of a Catskills tummler.

After 20 minutes, Tochterman put down the last storyboard and returned to his seat. He imagined himself being showered with praise and even pictured one of the dealers handing him the keys to a brand new Chrysler New Yorker.

"That was magnificent, Glen. We don't often do this, but the quality of that work and the panache you brought to the presentation was simply amazing. We want you to have this. We hope you like white leather with the red landau roof."

That's how well Tochterman thought it went. The dealers felt otherwise.

The lights came back up and a silence descended upon the huge conference room. Then Frank Tompkins, from San Diego, the same Frank Tompkins who torpedoed Riley's contract, a fireplug of a man with close-cropped hair and a hair-trigger mouth, pushed his seat back from the long table. The four steel legs of the chair screeched across the floor, gouging a good sixteenth of an inch off the beautiful 75-year-old hand-laid tiles.

He stood up, cleared his throat and when he was sure he had everyone's undivided attention, bellowed, "I don't know about the rest of you Asswipes, but I'm not sinking a dime of my money into any of this BULLSHIT!"

Frank sat back down. It was as if a bomb had gone off and the only sound that remained was the ringing in the ears. That ringing sounded a lot like...

"I'm not sinking a dime of my money into any of this Bullshit!"

Tochterman was relatively new to the business and had never been on the receiving end of such blunt client feedback. He simply took a deep breath and sat in his seat awaiting further instructions. The Bozell guys from New York, industry veterans, thought they had heard and seen it all.

Frank changed all that.

"I'm not sinking a dime of my money into any of this Bullshit!"

They fidgeted. Looked at each other.

And then Bozell's senior man, a smooth talking management supervisor who had worked on all the major automotive accounts, including Ford, Chevy, VW and even Jaguar, but who more importantly had gotten the practice of eating client poop down to a science, stood up.

"Frank," he said, "I want you to know that this is simply a work in progress. We're here to hear you out. To get your feedback. To make the necessary corrections that will make you happy. And move those Chrysler Plymouths off the lot. Make no mistake, Frank, your input is critical. In fact, because you have been so vocal on the matter, your input may be the most critical. I want you to know that we will marshal all the resources necessary within the global network of Bozell Advertising to deliver scripts that meet your exacting standards of excellence."

Frank, a seasoned car guy who was hawking used clunkers while this NY clown was still in diapers, flashed some teeth and then turned to one of the attendants clearing the lunch dishes.

"Honey, can you get me another Seagram's and soda?"

Weeks later, Glen Tochterman was on the set of a different Chrysler Plymouth dealership, somewhere in the heart of the Inland Empire.

The Coach Who Would Not Speak

The previous round of work died an inglorious death. And The-Almost-End-Of-The-Year Sales Event was pressing. So all the new work had to be redballed. There was no time for pre-approvals.

Instead of lazy poolside lunches and Beverly Hills coffee shop chitchats, Tochterman ate pizza at his desk, gave up weekends and rarely got home before midnight.

Still he was optimistic. And battle-hardened.

A little give, a little take, and Tochterman quickly learned how to dodge bullets and get scripts through the various levels of approval.

He had every reason to believe things were on the mend. And that he was going to come out of this ordeal with six or seven brand new television commercials, one of which might even be good enough for his portfolio.

That was the hope anyway.

Until after a lunch of poached Chilean Sea Bass, red beans and rice, and perfectly roasted plantains, Mr. Montalban turned to page two in the script, saw the copy about factory cash rebates and announced, "I'm not reading that."

He walked off the set, adding, "I'll be in my trailer."

Death on Mulholland Highway

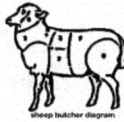

sheep butcher diagram

"Let's kill him," blurted Kathy.

"Let's kill this campaign and come up with something Mankowitz will actually buy so we can get the hell out of here. Is there any more coffee?" replied Maggie.

"What about a new twist on demonstrations? We can go old school and do a whole Volvo/BMW kind of thing," said Peter as he grabbed the last piece of pineapple, ham and cashew nut pizza from the greasy half-torn box.

Dave jumped on his case immediately.

"Dude, did you really do that?" Dave barked.

Peter tried to answer but his mouth was still trying to make sense of the cacophony of flavors that had been stuffed into it.

"Sawwwwy."

"You did this last night, too," said Dave as he pulled his fleece sweater over his soft, doughy belly. "We were creeping up on 1:00 A.M. and there was one box of Mushu Pork left. I might have wanted a bite of that."

Pete cleared his throat, "You said you don't eat after eight. You know you're trying to lose weight."

"I don't eat after eight on a regular night. At home. This isn't home, this...," using his big clubby hand to motion around the war room and the tired art directors and copywriters in it, "is not a regular night."

"Well, I can't keep up with your fluctuating eating habits," said Pete.

Dave rolled his eyes, secretly seething about Pete's voracious appetite and his rail thin physique. Adding, "If I ate like you, I'd look like me."

Before the bickering escalated, as it always did and it always would, Kathy seized the momentary silence.

"I'm serious, we should kill him. We should kill Mankowitz," she said, with a stare that left no room for doubt.

It got so quiet you could hear a chunk of pineapple drop.

The mood was markedly different a year ago.

They were all in France. At the Cannes Awards, advertising's version of the Oscars. Working as a small pod, they had produced a stunning integrated campaign for their automotive client.

It included a 60 second Super Bowl commercial about a little boy who travels with his parents on a science expedition to the Amazon. A torrential rainstorm tears through the jungle encampment and the boy is lost. The parents can never find the infant and he is raised by a pack of three-toed sloths.

Years later, the little boy is found and returned to his parents in Connecticut, where he has a difficult time readjusting to life at a normal pace. He walks slows. He talks slow. He even breathes slow. That is until the boy lays eyes on a beautiful black fastback with a 5.0 liter V-8 engine. His is magically reawakened by the need for speed.

Pitted against other Super Bowl commercials with tired celebrities, including Regis Philbin, Snoop Dogg and the Honey Boo Boo child, the whimsical spot easily captured the number one position in the all-important *USA Today* poll.

Sloth Boy became the darling of the Twitterverse.

Of course, there were a slew of integrated, brand-engagement follow-ups. A music video. A viral film. Even a live 24-hour webcam, where interested viewers could log on and see what Sloth Boy was up to.

It was all stellar top-notch work. And there they were at the Auberge Provencale, the oldest restaurant/inn in all of Cannes, to reap the Titanium rewards of their labor.

Dave pushed his bowl of *astoux et cie brun* towards Pete. "You've got to taste this dude. It's like a spoonful of sex."

"Is that a good thing?" Pete laughed.

Maggie was eyeing the Grand Marnier soufflé at an adjoining table and quickly snagged a waiter while the snagging was good.

"...and another bottle of the *Chateau Cabrieres*," she added while mauling the native tongue.

They were living large. And why not? Their client, Ted Kaplan, their happy client, the man who preceded Mankowitz, was seated at the table and was more than eager to foot the bill.

Ted had a keen understanding of their symbiotic relationship. If they were successful, he was successful. And the more meaningless industry trinkets they took home in their bag, the more cold hard cash Kaplan would be taking home to his wife.

He often told his marketing colleagues that he felt like a jockey who had been saddled on a thoroughbred horse. If he treated them right and fed them right, he could ride this horse straight to a Triple Crown.

"Champagne for the table," he shouted at the waiter. Then looking around the room and making a quick mental note of its relatively small size, he added, "...champagne for the entire restaurant."

Even Kathy, the most cynical of the group and the least likely to give in to the manufactured camaraderie, found herself lost in the moment.

The client wasn't done ordering.

"I also want a wheel of your stinkiest cheese. When we cut it open I want them to be able to smell it in Ireland."

Their incredible success with the Sloth Boy campaign was by no means their first. Working as a pod/team, they had produced legendary advertising campaigns, year after year.

In the relatively small world of advertising creatives, they were legitimate rock stars. But they never acted like rock stars. They didn't wear stingy brim Fedoras. They didn't sport funny designer glasses. And none of them, not one of the six, bore a tatted sleeve, an affectation that screamed mediocrity.

Though it's rumored while judging a One Show Awards Festival in Aruba, Pete, fueled by absinthe and pulsing reggae music, had a butterfly tattooed on his taint. For obvious reasons, no further inquiries were made.

Their success was rooted in meritocracy. They travelled the world. They stayed in the finest hotels. And ate the finest foods, because they produced. They came up with the breakthrough ideas that made Fortune 500 companies, Fortune 100 companies.

They labored under the belief, a naïve belief, that putting the best work on the table would always produce the best possible results. And for years, it had.

That is until they met Stan Mankowitz.

Stan the Man, only those directly under him accommodated that nomenclature, was brought in to replace Kaplan, who had been lured away by Nike.

Mankowitz had only been in the position for a few months, but had already made life a living hell for the five remaining members of the team. There had been six but Bruce, a short-tempered art director, couldn't stand to be in the same room with Stan. He made good on his threat and left advertising altogether; he invested in a coin-operated laundromat and was already making a mint with under-the-table cash income.

Stan Mankowitz was their problem. And Kathy, the untitled leader of the team had the solution.

"We have to kill him."

"You can't be serious. There's got to be another solution," said Maggie.

"I'm all ears," replied Kathy.

Pete chimed in, "Maybe we can get him fired?"

"How do we do that?" Kathy asked. "Oh wait, I know, we'll call the CEO."

"Yeah hi, you don't know me, I'm part of the creative team at your ad agency. And your new CMO is being very difficult. He doesn't like any of our ideas. He can't articulate a strategy. He depends on committees and focus groups because he can't make a goddamned decision. And his thinking is as thick as mud."

"Yeah, that'll work," said Kathy, who was no stranger to sarcasm.

110

"We're not the first creative team with a difficult client," offered Dave.

"No, we're not. Good point, Dave," conceded Kathy, who knew one of the best ways to persuade her cohorts was to give up some meaningless ground.

"But let's take a little inventory. It's 1:37 A.M. on a Tuesday night, I'm sorry a Wednesday morning. We've been holed up in this room for the past two months."

They were all nodding in agreement.

"Correct me if I'm wrong, but three weeks ago, Mankowitz gave us a 24 hour turnaround to see some new ideas. That was after we had shown him 167 storyboards."

For emphasis, she walked over and rested her hands on the stack of foamcore boards that had reached shoulder height.

"That was the same night Pete had planned an anniversary dinner with his wife," added Kathy.

"You had to cancel that dinner, didn't you, Pete?"

He just nodded.

"Did you make it up to her, Pete? Did you?" she said already knowing the answer.

Pete mumbled, "We're sort of going through a trial separation right now."

"Isn't that nice? I'm sure you'll smooth things out with her once we get a campaign sold, take it to focus groups in Toledo, Phoenix and Tampa Bay, re-do the idea, plow through hundreds of nights of cold pizza, shitty Chinese food and weak ass Costco coffee. Shoot the damn thing on a soundstage in Van Nuys and then spend another eternity re-cutting countless versions until Cecil B. Mankowitz approves one. Maybe two years from now. Does that sound right?" said Kathy.

Kathy looked over at Tim, who hadn't said a word all night. That wasn't unusual, Tim was the quiet type. And tended to do all his communicating with his pencils and markers.

He looked up at her and flashed her a quick glimpse of a drawing he had just sketched. It was Mankowitz on a crucifix. Tim smiled.

She could see the tide starting to turn.

"You're talking about killing another human being?" said Dave.

"No, I'm talking about killing Mankowitz. A conniving corporate ladder-climbing douchebag who is sucking us into his abusive little vortex of chaos, sweat and endless demands. It will not stop, unless we stop him."

Maggie jumped in, "We're art directors and copywriters, we're not murderers."

"Well, maybe we should be," said Kathy. "Did you read about that girl in Japan? She worked 54 hours non-stop on some banner ad until she keeled over on her keyboard. They're killing us. When are we going to fight back?"

"I don't want to get caught," replied Pete.

"Stupid, sloppy people get caught. We're not stupid. And we're not sloppy." said Kathy.

"Because I don't want to go to jail," said Pete.

Dave chimed in, "We're already in jail, Pete. We haven't left this room in weeks. They bring food to us, so we can keep working. And I hear HR is gonna put a stainless steel toilet bowl right there in the corner. Pretty soon we're all going to be watching you and your shy bladder try to pee in the bowl."

Pete interjected, "Ok, so our working conditions are less than ideal..."

"If your definition of ideal is being stuck in a North Korean Re-Education Camp," said Kathy, adding, "Hey, let's order out for more boiled carp."

"My point is, don't you think murder is a little extreme? Not to mention risky," Pete replied.

"Of course it's extreme. Of course it's risky. But you know who asked us to push the envelope and go bigger than big? Mankowitz."

Kathy grabbed a print out of an email the team had received from Mankowitz after reviewing the latest round of work.

"I didn't want to share this with you, but I'll share it now."

She cleared her throat in order to give it the right inflection, knowing that Mankowitz's words would make them squirm and wish it would all be over.

The latest round of creative was excellent. Some of the best work your team has ever done. Had I not known what you were capable of, I would have green-lit the work and hired the best production team on Earth to bring it to its rightful fruition. But I do know you. And I know of the tremendous creative firepower that your team wields, day in and day out. So while I love this work, and I wouldn't change a thing about it. I don't Love-love this work. I know how painful it can be to go back to the drawing board and stare at that intimidating blank sheet of paper. And I am kicking myself for making you do it. I would ask that you give this another shot. It's such a huge opportunity. If I had any helpful advice for you, it would be this: Scare me.

Make me nervous. Come up with an idea that is so big, so bold, that when I first hear it I will be on the verge of a heart attack. A wise man once said, without great risk there cannot be great reward.

"That passive-aggressive motherfucker!" shouted someone in the group.

The pitch, Kathy thought to herself, couldn't be going better.

"What do you suggest we do?" said Pete.

"I suggest we follow his instructions to a T," answered Kathy. Adding, "We should give him a heart attack."

The body language in the room changed. Crossed legs became uncrossed. Torsos slung back on beanbag chairs were now leaning forward. And Beats headphones, cocked with one ear open and one ear listening to bad electronica music, were now removed.

"I went online and read about Mossad, you know the Israeli CIA. Those guys are pretty damn clever. Did you know you could cause someone to have a heart attack just by slipping something in their drink? Or in their food? Hell, they figured how to induce a cardiac arrest just by having the victim touch a surface. Now that's cold."

Dave stopped her.

"Your entire scheme just went off the rails, Kathy."

"How so?"

"You did an online search? That's the first thing these forensics guys look for. That's CSI 101."

"Oh Dave. Sweet naïve, pizza-less Dave. Give me a little more credit than that, won't you?"

Death on Mulholland Highway

Kathy reached in her pocket and pulled out a jump drive.

"See this? This gives us access to a double-encrypted portal, an internal network within the internal network. We can do all our research, purchase any equipment and store any documentation in this walled off area that the cops would never, ever find. It's all buried beneath an accounts payable invoice from....(she pulls a small slip of paper from her back pocket)...February 28th, 1994."

The team never ceased to be amazed with her ingenuity.

"How did you manage that?" said Pete.

"I cut a deal with Kevin on the sixth floor," replied Kathy.

"IT Kevin?"

"That must have cost you a pretty penny," said Dave.

"Money is not the preferred currency of the 35-year old, manga-addicted computer nerd."

Maggie grimaced, "Ewwwwwwwwwww."

Kathy couldn't resist the softball set up.

"Let's just say I reformatted his hard drive."

"Stop," said Maggie.

Kathy continued pitching the plan. And each team member took a turn to play Devil's Advocate. Murder was not something they were willing to take lightly. But like a seasoned pro, Kathy ducked and weaved and bobbed. She had an answer for every question. And a contingency for every possible slip up.

By morning's light, they had all agreed. Stan Mankowitz must die.

The next few days were brutal. They spent half their waking hours concepting a new, breakthrough, award-winning campaign for the client. It was important to give the appearance of normalcy.

The other half of their waking hours was spent putting in place the apparatus of the client's demise. Making sure he would never enjoy the fruits of their labor.

As he did just a month ago, appearing on the *Ellen DeGeneres* show to revel in the success of a campaign he had nothing to do with. Mankowitz didn't even have the good grace to mention their names or the ad agency responsible for creating – in Ellen's words – "...the coolest advertising I've ever seen."

A price would be paid for this career-making snub, the ultimate price.

Indeed, the two efforts were intertwined. In another testament to Kathy's inventiveness, she came up with a campaign idea that would lay the foundation for their alibi.

In today's 360-degree world, every effort needs a viral film. To make their viral film, Kathy and her team would need lanyard making equipment, security guard uniforms and a recently killed beaver.

"The dead beaver," Kathy explained, "will provide the dried perineal glands. From which we can extract castoreum. The same fatty acid needed to make ricin. The ricin, combined with a powerful, but completely organic nerve stimulant, will first stun him and then launch his heart into a full blown myocardial infarction."

"Holy shit!" said Pete.

"I know," Kathy said calmly, "those Israelis know a thing a two about pulling off the perfect murder."

"No, Holy shit, I can't believe we're talking about taking a man's life and filling out purchase orders for a dead beaver."

Two weeks later, they found themselves seated with Stan Mankowitz in the Regency Room at the Beverly Wilshire Hotel for the annual Western Addy Awards.

As the presenters were on stage announcing the latest winner of the Rich Media 84 x 225 Digital Banner Ads, under 10K category and the tuxedoed servers were placing over-poached salmon in front of the attendees, Kathy leaned over and whispered something to Mankowitz.

"I have a present for you."

"For me?"

Stan loved being kissed up to. She inched towards his ear and purred.

"But I don't want the others to see me giving it you."

He understood completely.

"Give me the keys to your car, I'll leave it in the backseat."

He stealthily reached in his pocket and slid it under the table into her hand. While it was there he couldn't resist the urge to cop a feel of her inner thigh.

She took the keys and clenched her teeth into a smile, knowing that would be the last time he'd ever trespass there again.

Kathy excused herself from the table and made her way to the elevators, clutching the keys in one hand and a small vial of the weaponized beaver entrails in the other. She made her way down to P3 and spotted Tim, dressed as a parking lot Rent-A-Cop. Tim pointed out Mankowitz's 1987 Porsche 911, a classic sports car restored to near perfection.

Kathy couldn't help thinking every stitch of leather and every square inch of chrome on this beautiful machine was paid for by her team's blood, sweat and tears.

She opened the heavy door and eyed the burled wood of the manual stick shift knob.

She was in.

The belly of the beast.

"Out, out, damn spot," rang through her head.

She took several deep breaths to calm her nerves and steady her hands.

Fifty yards away, Tim stood guard. Making sure that no one saw what Kathy was about to do. Moments later he heard the thud of the door closing, followed by the door locking mechanism, followed by the clacking of Kathy's high heel shoes against the cement floor.

On her way back to the elevator she walked by Tim. He noticed her face was positively green. Not surprising, he thought, considering what had just transpired.

She returned to the table and her poached salmon had turned cold. Which was fine because she wasn't in the mood for eating. Her loss of appetite was contagious. With the exception of Mankowitz, no one was eating. Or talking.

The next day at the office was no better. The team gathered in their war room, which now seemed an appropriate moniker.
They pretended to work and did their best to avert eye contact with each other.

Pete said, "I don't feel well."

Death on Mulholland Highway

His stomach was doing cartwheels.

At 10:30 A.M., Brittany, their overly perky account coordinator, who was fond of surprising the team with cronuts and fresh-squeezed orange juice, brought something else. She held a print out of an email she had just received from the client.

"Oh my gawd, oh my gawd, Stan. Stan Mankowitz. He's dead!"

"What?"

"He's dead. They said he had a heart attack while driving home on Mulholland and his car went off the side of the road."

Pete sprinted to the men's room.

The war room, which was quiet before, was quieter now. They had killed the client who so often killed their work. Dave felt yesterday's lunch ~ he hadn't eaten since then ~ start talking to him. He exited quickly. Maggie followed, on the same path to the rest room. Tim took the news in stride and continued doodling on his sketchpad.

Kathy sat back in her beanbag chair, confused, wondering how life had led her to this.

A week later she found herself sitting on a wonky wooden chair inside the interrogation room of the Van Nuys Police Department, a place the detectives call The Box.

"We know about the online research. The Mossad websites," snapped the veteran homicide cop.

Kathy felt her breathing get difficult.

"We know about the security guard uniforms."

Her chest was getting tighter.

"And we know why you contacted the taxidermist for a dead beaver."

Kathy wanted to speak but no words would come out of her mouth.

"Oh yeah, your little friend Kevin, the IT schmuck, he gave it all up."

"Kevin? I don't know any Kevin," said Kathy, who figured denial was the best line of defense.

And added, "We showed Kev some pictures of what they'd do to his pretty little face at Chino Hills Correction Facility and he squealed like a pig."

Kathy started sobbing. The cop flipped a packet of tissues across the table to her.

The veteran detectives let it play out as it had played out in The Box a million times before.

"I didn't do it. We didn't do it. We had it all planned out. Every little detail. But when it came time to smear the poison...not poison...but you know...the stuff on the stick shift, I chickened out. I tucked my tail between my legs and got out of there. I didn't kill him. We didn't kill him."

"We know that."

"What?"

"We know. It's all on the security camera footage."

Security cameras! How stupid, Kathy thought, a rookie mistake.

"We know you didn't kill Stan Mankowitz."

"You do?"

"We also know who did."

"Who?"

The detective reached for his pocket and pulled out a hand-sized moleskin notebook. "Do you know this guy, Barry Hargrave?"

"Never heard of him."

"Yeah, he's an art director from Sherman Oaks, works at some immersive social media experiential agency. What the hell is an immersive social media experiential agency?"

"I don't have a clue," she said.

"Well, like you and your coworkers, he had a serious axe to grind with Mankowitz. He worked with Stan long before you guys. And he hated the man twice as much as you did."

He popped open a laptop computer and showed her some grainy video footage.

"That's Hargrave right there. Crawling under Mankowitz's car and cutting the brake lines. By the time poor Stan got up to Mulholland, that master cylinder was bone-fucking dry. He pumped the brakes and there was nothing left. Poor schmuck had a coronary and went right over the embankment."

"So...," Kathy stammered.

"So, while you researched a murder. Planned a murder. And walked right up to a murder...you didn't actually commit a murder. Besides, we already got a hump to pin this on. So go on, get out of here."

Kathy stood up, her legs wobbled a bit, but she managed to leave the police station under her own power.

That night, the team gathered in the war room, just as they had done a thousand times before. They bickered over soggy falafels and the last spoonful of spicy hummus.

And they got back to doing what advertising people do best, criticizing the work of other ad people.

"Cut the brake lines?" said Pete.

"What a bunch of amateurs," said Dave.

"Hacks. Total, social media hacks."

Weinblatt Goes to Germany

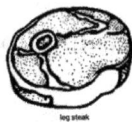

leg steak

Weinblatt Goes to Germany

Barry Weinblatt grew up in the shadow of the Holocaust.

His ancestors, from the prime Jew-harvesting fields of Belarus and Poland, boarded a steamer bound for America in the 1930's. And escaped the bloody hands of Hitler's henchmen.

But that didn't stop the Weinblatts from bearing a grudge. They were feverishly anti-German.

One Hanukah, Aunt Pearl flew up from Boca Raton. She came to the Weinblatts with itchy sweaters for the boys and a new toaster oven for the kitchen. It was the latest model from Braun, the same folks who perfected the crematoriums. It had eight different settings and could toast up to six pieces of bread or four large bialys from Bagel Oasis on Horace Harding Blvd. to absolute perfection.

It was self-cleaning. Self-adjusting. And self-sufficient. It was the Mercedes-Benz of toaster ovens.

When Al Weinblatt, Barry's father, returned from dropping Aunt Pearl off at La Guardia airport for her return to Boca, the miracle Braun toaster oven was immediately tossed from the 10th story apartment into the large dumpster below the window.

Volkswagen might have been the *People's Car*, but it was never going to be the Weinblatt's car. The same rationale applied to Porsche, BMW and Audi, though there was little chance that Al Weinblatt, a postal worker on a postal worker's salary could ever afford the gold standard of German engineering.

Similarly, Al Weinblatt was no fan of Henry Ford who had noteworthy Nazi sympathies. Nor would he drive anything from

Weinblatt Goes to Germany

General Motors, whose vague connection to the Third Reich remains a mystery.

That left the Weinblatts little choice but to drive a Plymouth, more specifically the Plymouth Fury, an automobile that broke down so often its name aptly described the mood of its owner.

Adamant about not spending any hard-earned dollars on products made in Germany, Al Weinblatt wouldn't even let Mrs. Weinblatt stock Bayer aspirin (made in Germany) in the house. In fact they would masochistically savor the pain of a throbbing headache, much the way every spring, Jews pay homage to the bondage and slavery of their ancestors by eating bitter herbs. Or gefilte fish. Or matza.

"A good headache makes a good Jew," Al Weinblatt would say.

None of that stopped Barry Weinblatt from interviewing with Goethe & Partners, a German advertising agency set on opening a satellite office in Los Angeles.

Goethe wanted someone with big brand experience. Someone who had collected a closetful of industry trophies. Someone who had grown tired of holding company politicking and dime-squeezing and was looking for a more entrepreneurial opportunity.

Check.

Check.

And check.

Barry Weinblatt had been in the service of some of the world's largest ad agencies. On both coasts. And he had done well by them. Winning awards, making clients happy and keeping their names well placed in the press. But his compensation always seemed one step behind.

Weinblatt Goes to Germany

The week after being named a Vice President, the Human Resources folks put out a memo that company cars would only be available to Senior Vice Presidents.

The day after his fifth year anniversary, the stiffs from Finance let it be known that company stock options would only go to employees with six years experience.

And 15 minutes after being named a Group Creative Director, it was announced that travel in Business Class would only be offered to Executive Creative Directors.

Goethe & Partners had reached out to Barry Weinblatt at just the right moment in his career.

Coffee at Starbucks led to drinks at the Mondrian, which led to a full seven-course meal at the Westside's exclusive Valentino restaurant. It was here that Dierk Goethe offered Barry Weinblatt the job of Chief Creative Officer of Goethe & Partners/Los Angeles.

Following the exquisite tiramisu, Barry signed the contract papers. Dierk shook his hand and dropped a bombshell on him.

"Excellent. Three weeks from now we will go back to Frankfurt to meet the team and from there we will take a train to Vienna to meet our client, Leviathan, Europe's best selling energy drink."

The tiramisu, which had previously gone down so smoothly, now clogged in Barry's throat. Years ago, while gallivanting across the continent with his girlfriend, Barry had successfully dissuaded her from a dreaded trip to the Fatherland.

"Let's swing south and check out the Algarve region of Portugal. I hear they have great sangria."

Weinblatt Goes to Germany

There would be no Iberian diversions on this matter. Like so many before him, Weinblatt was getting shipped off to Germany, whether he liked it or not.

"Welcome to Lufthansa, Mr. Weinblatt. May I take your coat?"

Yes you may, Barry thought to himself, eyeing this Aryan beauty and trying not to look too conspicuous. Before his ass even touched the First Class seat, which in comparison to Coach looked more like a couch, he was offered a cocktail, a meal and his own personal DVD player for his exclusive use throughout the 12 hour journey.

Maybe the *sturm und drang* was all for naught.

In his head, Barry could hear his father's admonition, "Get off the plane now. It's all a trick. They're flying you to a relocation camp deep in the frozen hills of Bavaria."

He settled into his seat and hoped to avoid all the possible nightmares one might expect from a transcontinental flight. To his delight there were no screaming babies. No loud talkers. And no repulsive aromas.

He once flew to London seated next to an old alcoholic woman who smoked a carton of cigarettes before boarding the crammed 767. To mask the tobacco odor she marinated herself in some cheap perfume she had just picked up at the duty free shop.

"Would you like a bag for the perfume, ma'am?"

"Oh no, I'm going to use the whole thing once I get inside the ladies room."

For eleven hours Barry gagged on the toxic bouquet of Marlboro's, Early Times Rye Mash and Drakkar for women. That flight was Barry's own personal Hell.

Weinblatt Goes to Germany

This time, Barry thought, he would allow himself the luxury of enjoying the moment. He leaned against the window and watched as thunderstorms rolled across the Atlantic.

In Frankfurt, Weinblatt was greeted by Dierk, who eagerly grabbed his bags and whisked him off to a Mercedes-Benz parked illegally in the white loading and unloading zone. Dierk swiped the ticket off the windshield, crumpled it up and stuffed it in the glove compartment where it joined a mound of other crumpled up parking tickets.

Convenience and expediency were of the utmost importance to a man as busy as Dierk. This reassured Weinblatt, validating his choice to go with a company that had money to spare for life's little inconveniences.

They tore off from the Frankfurt airport, heading north on Autobahn 648 towards Kronberg. The diesel engine roared to life and forced Dierk to raise his speaking voice.

"We will go to the hotel. You can shower, freshen up and change your clothes, and then we have the first of many meetings. We are all very excited to have you as our guest. And the newest member of the team."

Weinblatt leaned in over the stick shift to hear him. He didn't catch most of it. He only heard his new German boss mention something about a shower.

"We have a long day in front of us," Dierk shouted, "better get your energy up."

With that he reached to the cooler in the backseat and grabbed Weinblatt a frosty Leviathan Energy Drink. Barry didn't care for the taste, part grapefruit/part urine/part antifreeze, but had convinced himself he'd better learn to like it so he chugged it down.

And then, to appear like a company man, pounded down another.

They exited the Autobahn and were now on the outskirts of Frankfurt. It seemed a very rural setting for a Hyatt or a Four Seasons, but, Barry thought, when in what used be part of the Roman Empire, do as the Romans do.

What Weinblatt didn't know was that Dierk had something else in mind, something a little more special. The Mercedes turned off the main road and drove up a long windy narrow road, covered by a lush canopy of trees. The trees opened up to a large courtyard and Barry Weinblatt looked up at the Schlosshotel Kronberg, a Dracula-like castle built in 1893, exclusively for Empress Victoria Friedrich.

"Isn't it magnificent? Don't you love it?"

Weinblatt bit his lip.

What he would have loved was a junior suite at the Ritz Carlton, with wi-fi, a fully stocked minibar and an exotic assortment of authentic European hand lotions and aromatic skin conditioners.

Instead, the bellboy grabbed his bags and together they climbed up five flights of winding stairs to the narrow room with a single bed and a tiny window from which, he imagined, Rapunzel could let down her hair.

Weinblatt fumbled for some deutschmarks and tipped the grumbling bellboy. An hour later they were back in the Mercedes heading towards Frankfurt.

The office of Goethe & Partners was everything Weinblatt had imagined it to be. The angles were sharp and distinctive. The furniture was cold and uninviting. Dierk was particularly proud of the plexiglass couch that could also be turned into a coffee table. Not a dirty dish was left in the sink. Even the bookcases looked as if they had been under the watchful eye of a meticulous art director.

Weinblatt Goes to Germany

They had sectioned off a separate office for their new American colleague. This, Dierk explained, would be Barry's home away from home when he visited Frankfurt for his mandatory four times-a-year meetings.

"We hope we see you more often than that, Herr Weinblatt," he chuckled.

When the downtown Frankfurt office emptied out, Weinblatt thought he'd be going back to the hotel to unwind and recover from a monumentally long day. His new *hauptsturmfuhrer* had other thoughts.

Blessed with an uncanny sense of direction, Weinblatt knew they should be driving north towards the castle in Kronberg, but they were headed south towards Rodermark.

"Do you like schnitzel?"

"I do, if *schnitzel* is German for sleep," Weinblatt thought to himself.

The restaurant looked as if it hadn't changed in over 100 years. A quartet of men led by a man in *lederhosen* playing the tuba was on center stage. The stage was surrounded by a dozen large round tables, each seating 10 loud and rowdy Germans. The place was packed. A thick cloud of cigarette smoke hung just below the ceiling.

Dierk found his table where many of his good friends were waiting and eager to meet the newest member of his team. Weinblatt shook their hands and tried in vain to remember all their names...

Hilde
Albrecht
Gottlieb
Heinrich
Konrad
Manfred
Gitte

Weinblatt Goes to Germany

Ulrich
Petra
Ernst

It was like roll call at a Hitler Youth camp, Weinblatt could hear himself thinking.

He felt his energy waning and let out an involuntary yawn. Dierk had just the thing. He reached into his leather man-purse, where he always kept some extra Leviathan Energy Drinks. Despite his better judgment and faced with an evening with no end, Weinblatt downed the entire can.

As he forced a grin and made small talk with the other dinner guests, who all spoke perfect English, he felt a strange moistness in his lap. Oh no, he wondered, had this marathon of a day taken its toll on his bladder and released its wrath on his light khaki pants?

During a moment of jocularity, he pushed back the tablecloth for a more detailed examination. What he saw lifted him out of his seat.

A large black Rottweiler had been hiding under the table and was slobbering all over Weinblatt's lap.

The table erupted with laughter.

"That is Blitz. He is friendly. He is not going to bite you," said the dog's owner, a burly man in a 1940's era herringbone suit. Blitz's owner jerked the leash that was attached to a spikey metal collar that barely made it around the Rottweiler's thick, muscular neck. It looked less like it belonged on a dog and more like it was taken from a BDSM orgy.

"Who brings a 120 pound Rottweiler to a restaurant?" Weinblatt thought.

Germans do, he said to himself.

Weinblatt Goes to Germany

The schnitzel was surprisingly tasty. Perhaps the Ornithine, rumored to have been extracted from elephant scrotum, the active ingredient in Leviathan, had stimulated Weinblatt's appetite. In any case, he left the restaurant with a belly full of schnitzel, brats and the finest German beer ever brewed, east or west of the Rhine.

He'd sleep well tonight, he thought. It was one more miscalculation in a day full of them.

Back in Rapunzel's room, Weinblatt finally laid his head on the thin, inadequate pillow. He stared at the ceiling waiting for sleep to end the day that started more than 26 hours earlier. But as the FTC will attest, you can't sell an energy drink in America if it doesn't fulfill the promise of delivering extra energy.

Over the course of a day that spanned one ocean, two continents and seven time zones, the three cans of caffeinated Leviathan were kicking in. Add to that the incalculable effect of jet lag and you've got the recipe for one interminable evening.

Weinblatt fired up the Magnavox, hoping that some television would bring on some much needed slumber. Unlike his dinner company, they did not have the good grace to speak in English, rendering every show incomprehensible.

Moreover, the old TV did not have a remote control. Every change of the channel required a trip from his child's bed to the chest of drawers by the window, where all he could see was the pitch black of the treetops surrounding the castle.

His watch said it was 10 o'clock in the evening, his body said it was 10 o'clock the following evening. That's how long he'd been awake.

He knew that he had to counter the chemical imbalance that was raging in his gut so he did what any ad man would do, he put on some shoes and headed downstairs to the bar. Surely something

132

American and familiar, like Jack Daniels, would settle his unsettled nerves.

He stepped up to the bar and using the unspoken International Language of Thirsty Foreigners ordered a double shot of Tennessee's finest. Weinblatt did the math and figured it would take a six shots to overpower the powerful energy drink that was surging in his bloodstream. And because he didn't have to drive or be anywhere or even talk to anyone, he threw his American Express card on the counter and motioned for the bartender to keep them coming.

Though no one paid him any attention, he was now sufficiently soused and he began imagining the conversations at the bar were all about him. This, despite the fact that the only German words he knew were *Gesundheit* and *Hefeweizen*. Drunken neurosis is never pretty.

"Look at the size of that man's nose," he heard one woman whisper.

"We should put the Bolsheviks on a train and ship them back to where they came from."

"They eat gefilte fish and cut their own penises."

He stumbled back up the five flights of stairs and lay down on the bed again. He stared at the curved coved ceiling and wondered if he had made the right move. He tried reading himself to sleep but Weinblatt was an art director and more of a picture book guy. He cracked open the *Sky Mall* magazine he had swiped from the plane and read it from cover to cover. Backwards and forwards. He didn't think it was possible, but the *Sky Mall* magazine, deadly dull at 35,000 feet, was even duller at sea level.

The telephone rang. It was the front desk.

"Herr Weinblatt, this is your 7:30 A.M. wake up call."

The call was unnecessary and only served to irritate him. He'd have been glad for 40 winks but over the course of the last day and a half, he had none.

Dierk was waiting in the lobby for him at 9 sharp. He had prided himself on his punctuality. He greeted Weinblatt with a hearty handshake and wasted no time telling him of his plans.

"Ready for a big day, my friend? I want you to meet some of our vendors. We'll swing by the office for a PowerPoint presentation that I need you to polish. And later I have a little surprise for you. But first, let's get some breakfast. Sound good?"

"Sure," Weinblatt replied, "I was wondering if we could stop by a druggist first, I have a bit of an upset stomach."

He didn't want to tell his new boss of his dreadful night or that he was hung-over/jetlagged/just plain anxious. Fortunately, Dierk Goethe had just the thing for what ailed him.

"We don't need a druggist, we'll swing by my *mutter's* house. She'll fix you right up."

Mrs. Goethe, a stoic woman in her late 70's, returned from the bathroom with an unmarked bottle of white pills. She handed them to her son who reached in the fridge, pulled out a cold can of Leviathan and handed both to Weinblatt.

"Here, wash it down with this."

As he was gulping the mystery medicine with the undeniably powerful wake up juice, Frau Goethe took the opportunity to stroll down memory lane.

"I've never been to America. I hear it is very nice. But I won't go there. My brother Gerhard was killed by an American. In the battle of the Ardennes. New Year's Day, 1945. A mortar from the 30th Infantry

Division landed in Gerhard's foxhole. He was thrown 20 feet in the air. And was impaled on a splintered birch tree..."

The old woman stepped to the side so she could better examine the aquiline profile of Weinblatt's face. Dierk grabbed Weinblatt by the arm and rushed him from his mother's flat.

The pills, meant to calm his rumbling stomach, didn't. In fact, not knowing what he had swallowed only made him more nervous. And made paying attention during the day's business meetings damn near impossible.

Against all odds, he managed to keep his eyes open. Heading away from the office in downtown Frankfurt, Weinblatt steadied himself as he watched the wind ripple through the trees on their way north back to Kronberg. He also noticed that Dierk had missed the exit on the Autobahn and was delving further and further into the countryside.

The Mercedes had pulled up to a marina along the Rhine River. At the edge of the dock was a large party boat chartered for this special occasion. The entire company was aboard the boat and they were about to set sail on a fully catered river cruise that would pass by St. Goarshausen and the legendary Lorelei Rock on the Rhine.

According to Teutonic lore, Lorelei, a beautiful *fraulein* who had been betrayed by her lover, is sent to a nunnery. On her way to the convent she comes upon this magnificent rock. She vainly tries to climb the rock but falls to her death. Her ghost spirit continues to live there and now takes her revenge on unsuspecting river-goers by causing accidents and dragging the sailors down to the bottom of the river.

The *kinder-folk* love this story.

As the tour guide was retelling the tale and as the riverboat rocked back and forth due to the unusually choppy waters, Weinblatt leaned against the rail secretly hoping a large chunk of stone would fall away from the cliff and put him out of his 41-hour misery. But he would have no such luck.

"We go all the way up to Hammerstein before the boat turns around. And still have another three hours to go. Isn't this great?" said Dierk as he wrapped his arm around Weinblatt.

Then he reached into the pocket of his blazer and pulled out a silver flask.

"This was given to me by my Uncle Dietrich. He took it from a dead French soldier in 1917. The good war. Lovely, isn't it?"

Dierk held out two glasses, filled with chipped ice, and emptied the flask.

"Peppermint schnapps," he said forming a fist and waving it in Weinblatt's weary face, "make you feel good. Strong."

Then he topped off the schnapps with half a can of Leviathan energy drink, which was always handy.

"Minty Whale."

Weinblatt knocked back the drink and forced himself to smile.

In the circular driveway of the castle/hotel, Dierk had some parting words for his newest employee.

"Tomorrow we have a big day. I will pick you up at the castle at seven in the morning. We will go to the train station and then we will head down to Austria to meet the client. The train ride is magnificent. Mountains. Valleys. Little hamlets oozing with old-fashioned German charm. And you will love Vienna. Who doesn't love Vienna? Get a good night's sleep."

Weinblatt Goes to Germany

That was the plan. Surely, after all this time Weinblatt's body would cooperate and take him to the place he most desired, the land of sleep.

He shut the blinds to block out the light from a low hanging full moon. He undressed and left the clothes strewn about the floor. He slipped beneath the blanket and felt his body fall into the crater of the mattress that had seen better days.

And then he waited for Morpheus, the god of sleep, to whisk him away for a good nine hours before his trek to Vienna.

But Morpheus must have been waylaid by the siren song of Lorelei. After much tossing and turning, 10 minutes turned into 20, which turned into 30, which turned Weinblatt into an anxious mess.

He put his bare feet on the cold wooden floor and stood up. He felt dizzy. More concerning however, he felt a pounding in his chest. The pounding in his chest became a throbbing in his wrists. And his legs. He was suddenly aware of every nerve ending in his body.

He couldn't blink his eyes without thinking, "My eyes are blinking."

At 44 years old, he thought he was too young for a heart attack. But he wasn't too young, or too old, for a full-blown panic attack, something he'd never had before, but was having now.

He wanted to crawl out of his skin. Instead, Weinblatt bolted from the room whose walls seemed to be closing in on him.

The act of getting out of bed and getting out of the room soothed his frayed nerves. His breathing returned to normal. Even the clamminess of his skin began to subside.

He had the fifth floor of the castle all to himself and started to roam the deserted hallway, which easily measured the length of a football field. It looked less like the hallway of a hotel and more like the musty corridor of a museum. The walls were adorned with paintings from the Renaissance period. Along the walls were sturdy credenzas and glass bookcases chockfull of curios and charms, representing a thousand years of rich Teutonic history.

Weinblatt comforted himself with the thought that before the savages took over in the 1930's, Germany was the cultural capital of the world; breaking new ground in art, music, literature and philosophy.

He came upon a piece by Paul Delaroche. Painted in 1846, it was titled, *The Wife of Vernet on her Deathbed*. A haunting depiction of a woman, her mouth agape, on a love seat looking as if she had just overdosed on morphine.

Not a promising start.

Next up was a lithograph, done in 1918, by George Bellows, *Massacre at Dinant*. A shocking oversized piece that depicted the aftermath of a mass murder of 674 Belgian civilians killed by invading German troops.

Followed by Otto Dix's 1924 drawing, *Stormtroops Advancing under a Gas Attack*.

Then a bookcase full of knives. Long knives. Short knives. Curved knives. Straight knives. Smooth knives used for amputation. Serrated knives used for decapitation. Cleavers. Scalpels. Even pearl-handled, lady knives.

Twenty feet down the hallway was another bookcase, this one full of skulls. Old skulls. Young skulls. Baby skulls. Even wolf skulls.

And just beyond that another bookcase, this one filled with skulls that had been impaled by knives.

Everywhere Weinblatt looked there was death, carnage, bloodshed, and mayhem. A visceral reminder that no matter how much joy, laughter and beauty we are able to squeeze out of life, none of us are getting out alive. The Germans, it seemed, the original nihilists, made it a practice to go out in full-technicolor, Tarantino style.

Weinblatt felt his breathing get shallow again. And became painfully aware that his eyes were once again blinking. He went back to his room, pulled a chair up to the window and waited for the sun to rise.

When it did, he decided to tell Dierk Goethe what his body had been telling him all along: this was not the right job for Barry Weinblatt.

"I'm going home."

Between the jet lag, the chemical imbalance, and the onset of panic, the past 57 hours had been excruciating. But the silent, 30 minute drive to Frankfurt airport was even more painful.

Neither Dierk nor Weinblatt said a word. At the terminal, no handshakes or goodbyes were exchanged.

"Thanks, I'm really sorr..."

The Mercedes sped away.

Weinblatt passed on the complimentary champagne being poured by the flight attendants in First Class. An exquisitely beautiful Japanese woman sat next to him in 2C and smiled.

It would have been rude, and impossible, for him to refrain from exchanging small talk with the woman, particularly since she was so eager to talk. She reached in her purse to show him something.

"I was here on vacation. It's an amazing country, don't you think?"

"Amazing," he nodded.

"We visited Dachau, just outside of Munich."

He nodded again; he was somewhat familiar with the place.

"It was so touching. Let me show you the brochure."

He eyed the pamphlet.

"Next time you come back here, you really should visit."

That's probably not going to happen, Weinblatt thought to himself.

The plane veered south, leaving Germany, and crossed into French air space. Weinblatt took a deep breath, his eyelids sank and for the first time in three full days, he slept.

The next voice he heard was that of the pilot.

"Please fasten your seat belts and return your trays to the upright position as we begin our initial descent into the Los Angeles area."

The $45 Million Dollar Birthday Party

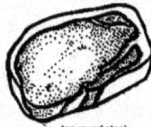

top round steak

"I'm writing it down," Goldman said into the phone, "a brown horsey piñata. Got it."

"Don't forget," his wife said into the phone for the thirteenth time, as if forgetting were in the realm of possibility.

"A brown one," she barked.

The next thing he heard was a click. Which was just as well. Goldman hated talking to his wife while he was at work. Particularly at this new job, working with Hat Rack, a boutique ad agency on the lower East Side.

Their offices once housed a woodworking factory that, not surprisingly, churned out hat racks. Out went the lathes and the ripsaws. In went the Mac Pro Towers, the Banksy posters and the single-serving espresso coffee makers. The office renovation didn't include any money for cubicles.

Goldman sat at the community worktable, an idea proffered by 21st century commercial interior designers, who now insisted on being called Experiential Office Anthropologists.

The Table was egalitarian. It eliminated hierarchy and promoted a more democratized environment. As a result, they claimed, ideas would be more freely exchanged, collaboration would skyrocket and creativity would flourish.

He didn't buy any of that.

Most of the staff had their noses buried in Zappos.com, never talked to each other, and never collaborated.

The $45 Million Dollar Birthday Party

The founders collaborated. Behind the closed doors of their offices.

The Table also obliterated any notion of privacy. So all these Hat Rack hipsters, with their funny designer glasses and $100 faux lumberjack shirts, knew Goldman was henpecked. That's why he tried to keep the communiqués with the wife to a minimum.

But as much as he hated the Table, he loved his new surroundings.

He was no longer employee # 26783, a tiny cog in the Big Ad Agency Machine. At Hat Rack, he was Goldman, the go-to-guy on sports, beer or anything that hinted of testosterone, which despite the excessive and well-groomed facial hair among the staff, was in very short supply.

Two weeks ago, the agency received an RFP for a new start-up cable network, the ACCN. A 24-hour sports channel devoted to the exciting Division One activities of the Atlantic Coast Conference.

Goldman's stock had never been higher. He was relishing this new opportunity.

Monday, 2:23 P.M.

Goldman and his team are four days away from the ACCN pitch. Winning a $45 million account will vault Hat Rack up to the next level. Loans will be paid off. Leases will be re-negotiated. And there will be a steady stream of revenue, meaning the boutique founders, headquartered in Europe, will back off on the pressure and grant the shop some much needed independence.

More importantly – at least to Goldman – a win like this could make his career. He could stop dilly-dallying with social media projects no one would ever see or use. And he could start making TV commercials, and eat at fancy sushi restaurants on other people's dime.

The $45 Million Dollar Birthday Party

He allowed himself to daydream a little; picturing himself at a state-of-the-art edit facility with all the latest technology at his command and a bevy of production assistants ready to bestow upon him the royal client treatment.

Yes, he thought, I will have one of those coffee drinks with the heart shaped foam carefully crafted on top.

The dream was within reach. And so was his cell phone.

It buzzed. Another text from his wife. His wife was first-born American. Her parents and her entire family were from Portugal. They were loud. And her text messages were loud. He knew if he ignored it, she'd be calling him moments, no seconds, afterwards.

Chocolate ice-cream cake. Big enough for 12 kids.

Got it, he texted back.

Friday was their son Levi's fifth birthday party. Which worked out perfect for Goldman, as his big ACCN presentation was Thursday night. He planned to work non-stop until the pitch and then take a well-deserved day off to celebrate with his son and a dozen furniture-busting kids.

The phone buzzed again.

No coconut sprinkles. The Levine kid is allergic and I don't want his mother getting on my case about some anaphylactic shock.

He should have been stunned that his wife knew the word 'anaphylactic' and equally surprised that she could spell it. But he wasn't; he learned a long time ago that she was a stickler for details and possessed the efficiency of a cyborg, built by other cyborgs.

Goldman made a mental reminder to himself: coconut equals castration.

The $45 Million Dollar Birthday Party

Tuesday, 9:13 A.M.

Goldman got to the office early. Early being a relative term. His co-workers wouldn't start strolling in until 11 or 11:30. They could be forgiven for their tardiness as they were all buzzing about the Hat Rack office well past midnight from the previous day. But he wanted to get a jump-start on the day and put the last polishing touches on the presentation.

Later, he would be showing the work to Hat Rack agency principal, Paul Henri, a serial entrepreneur who had his hands in everything from designer kale juicers to industrial flange distribution. Though he knew nothing about advertising, Paul Henri threw in with Hat Rack because he thought it would be "fun."

Henri knew the enormity of the pitch and wanted to satisfy himself that the Hat Rack team was headed down the right path. Goldman knew they were. He knew sports. More than anyone in the office.

They knew about designer lamps. Hair care products. And the best places in Manhattan to get *omakase*.

He knew about the 2-3 Zone, the crossover dribble, and the weak-side overload. In fact, he spent four white winters on the campus of Syracuse University. And even worked courtside as the man inside the Otto the Orange team mascot.

Goldman drew heavily on that experience to craft an entire campaign from the point of view of mascot characters. It was funny. It was insightful. And it was unlike anything ever done before.

He was sure Paul Henri would love it.

But Goldman still had a lot to learn about global advertising in the 21st century.

The $45 Million Dollar Birthday Party

Wednesday, 1:46 A.M.

The cleaning crew calls it a day. The mom and pop team of Guatemalan emigrants wring out the mops, empty the garbage and stash the cleaning fluids in the tiny janitor's closet. They would be back in 16 hours. But now they were going home to eat, sleep and recharge their batteries.

Goldman was not. He was there for the long haul.

He picked up two unsharpened pencils and tried tapping out a beat. This was futile since he didn't have a musical bone in his body. Never played an instrument. And couldn't carry a tune up a flight of stairs. A skillset that would have come in handy if he were to satisfy the request of his not-so-sports-savvy boss.

"We should do something with music," said Paul Henri earlier in the day.

"I like singing and dancing," he added. "We should do a campaign that feels like Rodgers & Hammerstein, Gilbert & Sullivan, or Sonny & Cher."

That's a bit effeminate, Goldman thought, not sharing the opinion with his slightly effeminate Belgian boss.

He couldn't see how a song and dance number would be an effective way to attract the target market ~ men who have never been to a Broadway show. And who would only consider going as a favor to their girlfriends or wives with the hope that their reluctant attendance would somehow result in oral sex.

Goldman also couldn't see how he could disobey the man who signs his paycheck every week and makes it possible to satisfy the demands of his other boss.

His phone began to vibrate, another text from Mrs. Goldman.

"Don't stay up too late. You need to get some rest for Levi's birthday party. The house is going to be full of screaming five year olds, including that Weinstein brat. And I'm not dealing with him all by myself."

It was almost two in the morning and Goldman felt the nerve just below his left elbow start to twitch. He looked down and could see the vein thumping. He tried to will it to stop. But the vein would not cooperate. So he watched it pulsate.

And as it did, he picked up on its regular beat. The beat turned into a rhythm. And the rhythm turned into song.

His musical muse had arrived.

Wednesday, 10:27 A.M.

"I like it. I like it a lot," said Paul Henri, who was not given to exuberance. "You have done excellent work here."

Goldman was relieved but had trouble keeping his eyes open.

"I thank you for doing this. To me there is nothing more important than commitment. I know you didn't want to do this. But you were a good soldier. I will not forget this."

Goldman felt his chest puff up.

"In fact, I want you to take the creative lead on the pitch. And insist you present both campaigns. This fabulous musical number and that thing you wrote with the funny costume men – the ascots?" said Paul Henri.

"The Mascots? Really?" Goldman replied.

"I know passion when I see it."

Goldman felt a surge of adrenalin and tried to rally the troops for the homestretch.

"Let's get going. We have a boatload of work to do before the pitch tomorrow."

Chai lattes were scooped up and laptops were folded as the Hat Rack team prepared to leave the conference room and man their battle stations for one last big push. The push that would net them a 45 million dollar account and transform them from a rag tag hipster boutique to a rag tag hipster boutique with a 45 million dollar AOR account.

But before they did, the Belgian had one little bombshell.

"One more thing and this is good news for all of you. The client called. They can't do the pitch Thursday, so they moved it to Friday. That gives us a whole extra day to get ready."

Everyone breathed a sigh of relief. Everyone but Goldman.

Wednesday, 4:58 P.M.

"Are you ready for this?"

Goldman pulled the phone away from his ear and mouthed, "I'm sure I'm not." Now his wife was calling, not texting. That couldn't be good.

"Sylvia Weinstein called. Wants to know if Max's little brother can also come to the birthday party. I don't remember the invitation having a plus one. Now we're gonna have two of those monsters running around the house, vomiting on the dog and wiping their asses with the living room curtains," said Goldman's wife before slipping into a Portuguese tirade.

The $45 Million Dollar Birthday Party

Goldman extended his chin, lowered his top lip and clenched between his two jaws, pressing harder and harder in an effort to distract his mind from the pain that was about to ensue.

"Did you buy the brown horse piñata yet?" she asked

"I've been a little busy."

"We're all busy, honey," she replied. "Levi changed his mind anyway. He doesn't want a horse, he wants a basketball. Did you write that down? A big, orange basketball."

"Got it."

"You should be proud. Levi knows how much you love basketball and he wanted to do it for you," she added.

When it came to his son, Goldman was like plumber's putty. She knew exactly how to push the Levi button and twist him up to suit her needs.

"And who knows how many of these Brooklyn JAPs are gonna drop their little princes at this party? You'd better get TWO basketball piñatas."

Goldman scratched out brown horse piñata on his To-Do List. And replaced it with orange basketball piñata. In parenthesis, he wrote 2.

Under that he wrote, Tell wife I can't make the party, followed by a series of oversized question marks.

Thursday, 12:21 A.M.

Goldman grabbed his thick, fleece overcoat, a red plaid shirt jacket that he simply referred to as *Schmata*. He told his co-workers he needed to get some fresh air.

The $45 Million Dollar Birthday Party

"*Schmata* and I are going for a walk, I'll be back in 20."

He had hoped a few minutes away from the Hat Rack office would help clear his mind. As he made his way down 2nd Avenue, he worked through all the permutations in his mind.

If he did the pitch he'd have a shot at winning a $45 million dollar account. These kind of at-bats don't come around that often. They're given less frequently to boutique shops that are usually consigned to below-the-line projects; useless mobile apps and websites visited by 138 people and then quickly tossed onto a digital landfill.

Pitching and winning this account, thought Goldman, could change the trajectory of his career.

On the other hand, the bigger, stronger slapping hand, she would never forgive him.

He missed birthdays 1, 2 and 4, because of pitches, presentation, re-pitches, focus groups, whatever the business demanded. He argued successfully that Levi would never remember those birthdays anyway, so his absence was never an issue. She, of greater foresight, countered that while Levi will never remember those special occasions, neither would he.

She was good with a knife.

Friday, 10:35 A.M.

Maria Goldman, still acquainting herself with American customs and their ungodly fascination with sports, led Goldman to the backyard to show her handiwork.

"I know you've been working really hard lately and I'm so happy that you took the day off for Levi's birthday party, so I already hung the piñatas."

The $45 Million Dollar Birthday Party

Goldman looked up and saw two orange *papier-mâché* basketballs hanging from the limb of the old oak tree in the backyard of their tiny Williamsburg home.

"I ran out of string, so one hangs lower than the other."

He stared at the pair of lopsided balls and knew right away that Paul Henri would soon have his.

He called the office and spoke with Patti, the Hat Rack receptionist. Feigning a scratchy throat, he explained to Patti that he would not be coming into the office that morning. And the team would have to do the big pitch without him.

Patti, an underpaid office temp with no skin in the game whatsoever and completely unaware of the magnitude of Goldman's absence, shrugged her shoulders and said, "Fine."

An hour later, the boys arrived at Levi's fifth birthday bash. There was screaming. There was yelling. There was bickering. And Goldman loved every minute of it. He managed to compartmentalize the moment and banish the worries of work to a distant corner.

Levi pulled on his dad's shirttail and made him sit next to him while they opened the presents.

Levi saved a seat for Goldman at the table for the cutting of the birthday cake.

Levi and his dad made funny faces for the camera.

Maria Goldman tied a blindfold around Max Weinstein's oversized head. He took the bat and started swinging wildly for the orange basketballs. Possessing all the athletic ability of a rhododendron, Max missed. And missed again.

151

The $45 Million Dollar Birthday Party

Max's little brother didn't have any better luck. Nor did any of Levi's friends, who seemed destined for MIT more than the MLB.

The front doorbell rang. Goldman handed the piñata string to his wife. He opened the front door of his modest Brooklyn townhome. It was Paul Henri.

"You disappoint me."

He fixed his pale grey eyes on Goldman and said nothing else.

"You drove all the way out to Brooklyn to say I disappoint you?" Goldman replied.

"No. I also want you to know that we will show your work in the pitch. And if we don't win the account I will fire you."

"Fair enough." Goldman replied.

"And if we do win the account, I will still fire you."

Paul Henri returned to his black Lincoln Town Car and drove off.

Goldman shut the door, took a deep breath and returned to Levi's birthday party.

He marched to the backyard and without saying a word; he took the bat from Howie Rothstein. He wound up and with a quick snap of his torso, his shoulders, his arms and his wrists, hit the orange basketball with the full weight of his Louisville Slugger.

Before anyone could react to the sudden spray of airborne candy, Goldman reeled back and laid another mighty blow on the other ball.

He kept smacking the two piñatas until the suspended *papier-mâché* basketballs were nothing but pulp.

The $45 Million Dollar Birthday Party

Bite size Milky Ways, Snickers, Hershey Kisses and Almond Joys covered the tiny yard from end to end. Amidst all the squealing, Goldman went back inside the house, poured himself three generous fingers of Maker's Mark and sat in his leather recliner. And stewed.

Two Weeks later

Representatives from the ACCN awarded the account to BBDO.

With one stipulation.

They liked the thinking and creative presented by Hat Rack and requested that the writer of the Mascot campaign be hired immediately and put in charge of the account.

Goldman is shown his new office, with a stunning view of the East River.

He doubles his pay. Gets a signing bonus. And inks a multiyear contract with an ironclad clause that in addition to the 15 paid holidays all BBDO employees are entitled to, he will be given one additional day off every year – the day of his son's birth.

He never missed another Levi birthday party.

A Proxy War in Midtown Manhattan

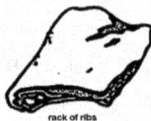

rack of ribs

A Proxy War in Midtown Manhattan

Fishman was fond of saying, "Less meetings, more work."

And so it was with great reluctance that he agreed to get on a redeye and leave the comfort of his home in Culver City, California for a few nights at the way-too-hip SoHo Grand in Greenwich Village, where rooms are often no bigger than closets and bottled water requires some light loan documentation.

This trip was particularly painful for Fishman as he was sent to receive the results of test marketing on a campaign he and his partner had given birth to more than 11 months ago. He had to refer to flash cards to remind himself of what he had written.

Long gone were the magical days when a creative team would show potential new work to a Vice President, who would show it to his wife, who would suggest changing the color of the car, who would then see her correctly colored automobile in a commercial running on television in a matter of weeks.

The process, once unwieldy but manageable, had become an interminable foot race. At one time getting work produced required the determination of a marathon runner, but now it necessitated the maniacal madness of someone willing to punish their body for a 100-mile ultra-marathon.

Fishman was not built for marathons. He didn't enjoy walking to the mini-mart for a half-gallon of milk.

His campaign had been tested in Omaha, Des Moines and Little Rock. The kind of places that would surely be hip to his brand of urbane cleverness and humor.

Of course it would have been nicer, and perhaps more telling, had they been testing finished commercials.

But these were not the miniature films he and his partner had envisioned. With real actors and actresses. Directed by a professional with an eye for nuance. Thirty seconds of well-crafted celluloid that could teach the clowns from Hollywood a thing or two about storytelling.

Instead, they had carted out poorly drawn animatics, which are, not surprisingly, exactly what they sound like: cheap cartoons, set to even cheaper needle drop music.

So the "work" they were showing the quickly assembled focus group of plumbers, housewives and fig farmers, who had agreed to give up an evening of their lives for fifty bucks and bad lasagna, was not ideal, to say the least.

As if that were not demoralizing enough, the purpose of today's meeting at the headquarters of FutureQuest™ was a deep dive into the results of Quantitative Copy testing. It is during this rigorous phase that, according to the FutureQuest™ brochure, "our marketing scienticians meticulously review and quantify copy ensuring maximum marketability and optimized persuasiveness across the full spectrum of human behavior. And guarantee the sustainability of a functioning marketing eco-system."

Fishman possessed a Masters Degree in Comparative English Literature, but could not make heads or tails of the FutureQuest™ credentials package.

From the pictures, he did notice they had a comfortable looking red couch in the reception area, where, between briefings, he hoped he might be able to steal away some shuteye.

His bemusement was not just reserved for FutureQuest™. There were hundreds of similar research companies making similar, if not grander claims of "changing the market landscape and delivering paradigm shifting results."

For one thing, the commercials he and his partner had created were for Coca-Cola. A few more million gallons of brown fizzy water might be sold, but Fishman doubted any landscapes were being changed. Or any paradigms being shifted.

Moreover, he failed to see how laymen, with no schooling or expertise in brown fizzy water marketing, just common people lured by the promise of free M&M's, would have anything meaningful or constructive to say about a piece of communication that had successfully run the gauntlet of a multi-tiered corporate hierarchy.

As testing went, these manufactured viewing conditions were nothing like the way people actually saw TV commercials. Or, if nature called, didn't see them. Had any real scientists been in the vicinity, the results of these "tests" would have been tossed in the same circular file reserved for Flat Earth arguments.

None of that seemed to deter the genii at Coke.

They swore by testing and counted on Fishman to heed the exceedingly expensive counsel of FutureQuest™ and make the necessary adjustments to exponentially expand brown fizzy water consumption.

Fishman could see he was running late for the debriefing. The redeye got in late and he arrived at the hotel at 9:30 A.M., just as most business folks were leaving. He thought he'd grab a few hours of sleep before the 1 P.M. meeting uptown and called the front desk for a late morning wake up call. The concierge jotted down the request and then promptly spilled his haute bottled water on the slip of paper, rendering it indecipherable.

As a backup, Fishman thought it would be wise to set the alarm.

However, as is often the case in trendy NYC hotels, the fashion-friendly alarm clock was designed by some Gehry-wannabe uber-minimalist. It had one button and no display. Fishman spent 20 valuable minutes trying to make sense of the white plastic orb, but couldn't.

Unshaven, tired and not at all happy about his situation, Fishman hailed a cab just off Canal Street. The sign on the door clearly read, "Non-smoking vehicle."

The driver of the taxi clearly didn't read English. He used one cigarette to light the next.

He pushed his way past the blue haze, barked out his destination and looked over at the medallion identifying the driver, Mohammed ben Abdullah. Gasping for oxygen, Fishman gauged the man's mood and decided against agitating the apparently angry man any further.

He cracked open the rear window and stuck his head out for precious oxygen.

Using his masterful skills of deduction, Fishman concluded that the bearded driver Mohammed was in his late 40's, probably a recent immigrant from North Africa or the Middle East and, in all likelihood, not an ardent follower of the Maccabee Basketball team.

At 8th Avenue and 15th Street, those suspicions were quickly confirmed.

As the light turned green, Mohammed was abruptly cut off by a yellow school bus on the left. Had it not been for some quick foot work, the kind of instinctive muscle memory that usually takes NYC hacks years to develop, Mo would have driven headlong into the back of an eight ton garbage truck that was still patrolling the north side of the Meat District.

A Proxy War in Midtown Manhattan

But he didn't. He slammed on the brakes, spun the steering wheel and then instantaneously accelerated, executing a geometrically impossible arc that saved their lives.

It was a close call.

Fishman looked out the window, spotted the Hebrew lettering on the side of the crusty, rotting school bus and knew this was not going to be good.

He slid over in his seat, poked his head out the driver's side and saw the bus was sardine-tight with Hasidic boys. Long curly *payos* sprouted from every window, from the front of the bus to the back; framing laughing faces that seemed to be mocking the Egyptian/Libyan/Yemeni/Algerian/Saudi cab driver.

The light turned red at 19th Street and Fishman's cab pulled up to the crosswalk, neck and neck with the school bus. Mo looked up at the driver, an older Hasid in his 50's, with a greying beard but a headful of bright orange hair tucked under a white *kippa*. Like Mohammed, he had little concern about the detrimental effects of second hand smoke. A lit Marlboro dangled between his snarling lips.

As young Chelsea hipsters navigated the walkways, a fiery flurry of Semitic slander filled the air. Mohammed hand cranked down his window – that's how old the taxi was – and shouted something indistinguishable in Arabic. The words might have been meaningless but the tone was unmistakable.

Rebbe Carrot Top responded with some choice Yiddish words of his own.

"Gai kaffen afen yam."

Which literally translates as *Go shit in the ocean*. Fishman recognized this as a variation on a phrase he often heard his father use.

A Proxy War in Midtown Manhattan

"Gai kaffen hoist." Or, go shit in your hat.

This, he found out later, was the curse preferred by residents of the South Bronx and Queens, where he grew up.

Angered Brooklynites opted for, *"gai kaffen ya ziwp"* – Go shit in your soup.

And inhabitants of Manhattan often used the more erudite, *" Gai kaffen ya bibliteck"* – Go shit in your library.

The cursing was accompanied by much spitting, which is unavoidable given the phlegmy sounds and inflections of both Yiddish and Arabic.

The light turned green and Fishman's cab darted out in front of the lumbering bus that looked like a holdover from 1959. Mohammed wasted no time cutting off the Hasid and his brood of cheering children. At 22nd and 8th the two vehicles came within inches of each other, pleasing both delirious drivers who were now under the influence of adrenalin and 1400 years worth of unresolved Abrahamic hostility.

Fishman found himself in a bit of a pickle.

He had no particular love for the Hasidim. He didn't care for their misogynistic patriarchy. Never understood their odd *shtetl* habits, including their refusal to turn a light switch on Saturdays or, apparently, take a bath or shower on the other days of the week. And then there was the business of Hasidic couples having sex through a hole in a bed sheet.

What kind of God commands his followers to ruin perfectly good bed linens?

Nevertheless, these were members of *his* tribe. Albeit fringe members who bred like rabbits. Their inordinately large families never had enough bedrooms or bathrooms, but for some ungodly reason their houses, or apartments, had two unexplainable kitchens, one for meat and one for dairy.

In any case, he'd have a hard time rooting against the home team.

Conversely, there was angry Mohammed, who made a habit of pounding his well-calloused fist on the dashboard of the old cab for every perceived slight. The vinyl on the dashboard had long ago been covered up with layers of grey, dirty duct tape. Despite being beaten into submission, the duct tape gave the taxi some much-needed structural integrity.

It would be easy to root against this man who seemed to have a scowl surgically implanted on his face, but Fishman found himself in the backseat of his cab, and consequently, at the total mercy of this New York City-licensed *jihadi*.

After a series of green lights, the Hasid built up a head of diesel-fueled steam and passed the cabbie on the right. The taxi swung to avoid the oncoming vehicle and cut off a bike messenger. The bicycle jumped the curb at 29th and 8th and took out a corner salesman peddling chocolate diamonds and fake Rolex watches. The goodies splayed out on the sidewalk. Savvy New Yorkers, keenly aware they had no value, stepped over the shoddy jewelry and timepieces and went about their business.

At 33rd Street the lights turned red. And, as it so often happens 6,000 miles away where Northern Africa meets the Asian continent, the indecipherable Semitic verbal parrying began again.

The door on the bus swung open, so the driver would have a clearer view of his Arab adversary. Words with a lot of 'ch's' and 'sh's' were exchanged.

Then came the falafel.

And the hazelnut mocha.

A Proxy War in Midtown Manhattan

It happened so fast, Fishman couldn't tell who initiated the firefight. He only knew that a half-eaten lamb *shwarma* sandwich was lobbed at the bus. And a full, grande sized coffee had been splattered across the windshield of the cab.

The light turned green and Mohammed hit the accelerator and turned on the wipers at the same time. Fishman got splashed with a wave of cold coffee. Between the cigarette smoke and the hazelnut, he now smelled like a Tunisian *shisha* bar.

A slow moving FedEx truck in the left lane gave Mohammed an opportunity to dart in front of the school bus. He wasted no time jetting out into the clearing. Then, with the skill of Mario Andretti, he darted back in and, in a near suicidal fit, slammed on the brakes. Fishman could hear the loud screeching as the rickety school bus was forced to do the same. He could imagine a flock of unbuckled Hasidic boys falling like bowling pins.

A moment later, as if by some Hanukah-like miracle, the bus flew by on the left side. Fishman looked out the window and saw a lone curlicue of black hair dangling off the corner edge of a window.

The spiral of long black hair was not attached to the child who grew it.

At 51st Street, construction crews had been called out to patch a busted water line. Orange cones had been laid along 8th Avenue, funneling all the northbound traffic into two lanes. The high-speed mêlée had been reduced to a simmering slow crawl. Again, not unlike their counterparts on the other side of the planet.

The cab would scoot up a foot or two and Mohammed would curse the Hasid.

The bus regained the edge and the rabbi retaliated with a few choice words and hand gestures of his own.

162

A Proxy War in Midtown Manhattan

Fishman looked up at the street sign and noticed he was at 52nd, just 5 blocks short of his destination.

He also noticed the legless veteran he'd seen at 46th street had already passed them. The meter read $17.85 and Fishman figured a $20 would cover the fare as well as a tip for the near death experience. He stuffed the bill through a hole in the plexiglass divider that barricaded the front seat from the rear. And with the cab still inching forward, lunged safely out onto neutral land.

He stepped onto the sidewalk, breathed a sigh of relief and removed a garbanzo bean that got lodged under his collar.

The receptionist at FutureQuest™ was happy to see Fishman. The feeling was not mutual.

"They're waiting for you in the Enterprise Conference Room."

Fishman dragged his carry on luggage, his backpack and his laptop down the hallway and seriously considered turning on his heels and making a mad dash back to La Guardia airport.

Fishman had a knack for reading a room and he knew the second he walked into the conference room, packed with waiting FutureQuest™ executives, this nightmare of a day was only going to get worse.

"Mr. Fishman," said the meeting leader, "glad you could join us."

Fishman replied, "You didn't have to wait for me."

"You are the writer of this campaign. You're the only one who can fix the many issues with the spots. It seemed pointless to start without you."

Issues, thought Fishman. Governments have issues, dysfunctional marriages have issues, psychopaths have issues, TV commercials about brown fizzy water don't have issues.

A Proxy War in Midtown Manhattan

For the next hour and a half Fishman listened as the FutureQuest™ scienticians dissected the work.

With a stunning, well-polished PowerPoint presentation, they noted the work achieved high scores for Memorability and Entertainment Value, but fell far short on Authenticity (79), Core Value Reflection (73) and Persuasability™ (68).

"Our acceptable benchmark is an 83."

Fishman had no idea what any of that meant. Nor did he have any clue how to bump up those miserable scores. With several Coca-Cola clients attending, he wisely decided not to go on the defensive. He simply smiled. Fidgeted in his seat. And took the verbal beating he so obviously deserved.

Before leaving the debriefing, Fishman put everyone at ease.

"I want to thank you for this valuable feedback and let you know that I've already begun hatching ideas that will address these significant issues to everyone's satisfaction."

Business cards were slid across the conference table. Post-meeting pleasantries were exchanged. And Fishman made a beeline for the elevator.

As he exited the building he spotted a Ray's Pizza on 57th Street. And relished the opportunity to decompress, enjoy some downtime and put some New York nourishment in his body.

"Can I help you, sir?"

"Yeah, I'd like two slices."

"Any toppings?"

Fishman looked up at the menu board.

A Proxy War in Midtown Manhattan

"Yes," he said, and in a defiant nod to the crazy Abrahamic adventures that brought him to midtown this fine afternoon, "I'll have one with the pork sausage. And the other with Canadian Bacon."

Pleased with his decidedly un-kosher and un-halal pizza topping preferences, Fishman went one step further, adding, "And throw some extra cheese on top of that meat."

The guy behind the counter had no idea why that brought such a smile to Fishman's face, but it did.

"Anything to drink?"

"A small Coke," Fishman replied instinctively.

"You know what, I hate Coca-Cola, make it a Pepsi. Large."

Redemption in Guanajuato, Mexico

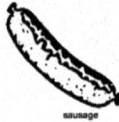
sausage

Redemption in Guanajuato, Mexico

In 1983, Meehan, Carter and Flears was the largest advertising agency in all of Los Angeles. Successful, laid back and the first to institute Casual Dress Fridays. At the end of any given week, it wasn't unusual to spot 100 different types of Hawaiian floral shirts drifting through the hallways of their sleek high-rise offices in Westwood.

MCF had a national car account, so unlike other satellite offices they were relatively untethered to the mothership in New York City. Moreover, because they were winning awards, the mucky mucks in Gotham were more than happy to leave MCF alone, collect the checks and falsely share in the glory.

And there was plenty of glory to go around. The creative department featured a deep bench of industry all-stars. At the yearly Belding Awards Show, the team from MCF would need a wheelbarrow to cart home all the awards they had collected.

If ever an agency were running on all 8 cylinders, in 1983, it would have been Meehan, Carter and Flears. Ironic, considering the car company they represented trafficked in 4 cylinder bangers that could squeeze every mile out of an overpriced tank of gas.

Back at the agency, each year's bounty was proudly displayed in a trophy case that sat in the 7th floor reception area. Visitors to the Wilshire Blvd. office could not miss the bevy of shiny silver bowls that threatened to crash through the shelves, now bowing, under the enormous weight.

A new display case had been ordered to accommodate the expanding collection. It was up to Tim and Dave, the mailroom clerks at MCF, to assemble the new case on the loading dock, far from the privileged divas in the creative department.

Redemption in Guanajuato, Mexico

Tim Jenson had been with MCF for over a year now. As most can tell you, a year as a mailroom clerk is like seven years as a mailroom clerk. This was particularly true for Tim, who had a Master's Degree in Fine Arts from Notre Dame University.

Little did Tim know that a year from standing under the outstretched arms of Touchdown Jesus and listening to the awe-inspiring commencement speech by a soon-to-be presidential candidate, that he, a graduate with an extensive knowledge of photographic lighting and 18th century water color paintings, would be schlepping boxes, stacking mailing tubes and keeping a close eye on the vertical filing cabinets.

This was not the world he or his parents, now down $30K, had envisioned at all. Tim was convinced the only thing more degrading than unemployment is underemployment.

"Which one is the damn supporting bracket?" he said looking over the assembly illustrations, "I think these directions were written in Mandarin."

With all the awards, and the subsequent growth at the agency, it was impossible for one mailroom clerk to attend to all the minutiae. Particularly when Tim found himself less and less an employee of MCF and more and more like a personal valet to Bill Wentworth, the head account guy on the $250 million car account.

Wentworth was an old-timey Detroit guy. He favored plaid suits, polyester, a comb-over and stinky Robusto cigars, Cuban, which were only sold underground at a secret tobacconist in Korea Town.

Wentworth would go through two cigars a day. This was a less enlightened time when executives were permitted to smoke in their offices. Even if the powers that be had outlawed the practice, Wentworth would have gleefully ignored them.

He had the car account in his back pocket. And for him, that was a license to steal.

"Tim, I need you to get in the car, head down Olympic and pick me up another box of those Don Domingo's."

"But Mr. Wentworth, Mr. Meehan (the agency president) has me clearing out these old files."

"What's your point, son?"

If it wasn't cigars, Tim was sent to retrieve Wentworth's dry cleaning, refill his eczema ointment prescriptions or drop by his house in Long Beach to make sure Mrs. Wentworth didn't leave the panini-maker on.

Tim was thrilled when some extra money showed up in the operations budget and the agency decided to add a second mailroom clerk. Let somebody else serve that pig, he thought, I have two college degrees and can identify 75% of the paintings at the Uffizi Museum in Florence.

The first applicant to be Tim's new partner was a UCLA transfer student who had come to the states from China. Tim didn't pass on her because of her cloying attitude. She was a couple of soba noodles short of five feet tall and weighed little more than a large wombat. When furniture needed to be moved -- and the prissy writers and art directors, always searching for the best *feng shui*, were constantly requesting to have their furniture moved -- he knew she would not be of much assistance.

The second applicant, Wayne, certainly had the muscular arms and legs for the job. Unfortunately, they were covered with homemade tattoos, with ink the prisoners at Folsom had learned to fashion from charcoal and used motor oil. Wayne had no interest in advertising, but his parole officer had sent him on every possible job lead.

Redemption in Guanajuato, Mexico

Dave Lang was the third and final candidate.

Like Tim, he was a recent college graduate.

Like Tim, he moved to Los Angeles to get into the entertainment business, anything in entertainment, including advertising, the streetwalking, dimwitted stepchild of the entertainment business.

Like Tim, he had a mischievous streak, though in Dave's case it was slightly more volatile, slightly more dangerous. The two hit it off immediately. Tim wanted to hire Dave. He shut the door to the mailroom in order to whet his appetite.

"...Free coffee, free parking in Westwood and lots of hot chicks work here," he whispered. Adding, "I'm also in charge of stocking the mailroom, paper, file folders and envelopes and such. You wouldn't believe what some of these salespeople will do to get some of that business."

Dave smelled a good story coming on.

"Three months ago, this new rep shows up from Precision Paper. She's wearing a tight white blouse and an even tighter grey skirt."

Dave leaned in.

"Did I mention she had on heels? High, high heels?"

"Black, with red painted toenails?" asked Dave, who wanted the whole picture.

"I tell her, we already have a reliable supplier of hanging collapsible file folders and that if I suddenly switch to a new vendor, my boss will get suspicious."

"Would he?"

"Hell no. He's got more important shit to worry about than where I buy the company's paper clips. But she doesn't know that," said Tim. "So now, she has to sweeten the deal."

"Did she sweeten the deal?"

"It doesn't get much sweeter, if you catch my drift?"

"I do catch your drift. Tell me about the company's dental care."

Tim and Dave got along famously.

Dave was thankful that, after a year and a half out of college, he finally had a foot in the door. This meant an end to the constant nagging from his parents, who were never happy with his interest in writing and had hoped he would pursue a promising career in something more solid, like chartered accountancy.

"There's good money in chartered accountancy," said Dave's dad. Better, he thought, than something soft, like writing.

Tim didn't have the heart to tell Dave that clerks never go from the mailroom to the creative department. Never. He knew once people saw you as a minimum wage errand boy, they would always see you as a minimum wage errand boy.

Nevertheless, he was happy to let Dave cling to such nonsense. Misery loves company. And in Dave, Tim now had someone who could share in the misery of Bill Wentworth.

A few weeks into the job, Dave stormed into the mailroom with an orange in his hand, purchased from the overpriced snack shop in the lobby of the building. He flicked open his Swiss Army knife and cut it into quarters. He squeezed the citric juices all over his hands, furiously trying to remove the awful stench.

"Fucking Wentworth," said Dave.

"What happened?" said Tim.

"He calls me in. Tells me it's Bring Your Kids into the Office Day. Then shows me the remnants of his kid's lunch. Seems his little princess is violently allergic to seafood. She carpet bombed his entire office with half the cast from *The Incredible Mr. Limpett.*"

"Why didn't he call the office cleaning crew?"

"I asked him the same thing. Then he explains to me how he's had several altercations with Flacco the Janitor."

"Altercations, really? A man of your warmth and incredible likability has had altercations?"

"You said that?" asked Tim.

"In my head I said that," replied Dave.

"Fuck Wentworth!"

Tim fought back the *schadenfreud.* And took silent joy that he was not the one scrubbing vomit off his hands or from under his own fingernails. Tim could also see his partner was quickly becoming disenchanted. Smelling like day-old, predigested lobster roll wasn't listed in the job description. He knew he had to cheer Dave up. And fast.

"Let's open some confidential memos."

It would be 10 years before computers started popping up on desktops. And another five after that before employees could instantly correspond with each via the Internet. And careers could be ended with an errant Reply All.

In 1983, secretaries talked to other secretaries, the way middle managers talked with other middle managers, and the way vice presidents talked with other vice presidents: they wrote memos. Some short. Some not short. And some not meant for prying eyes. Those were stamped in bold red ink.

"Do Not Open."

"Confidential."

"Private."

"Go Away."

Of course these exhortations had the reverse effect. If any memos were to be read, these were at the top of the reading list. And the powers that be hardly made it difficult to access the forbidden fruit.

In the 19th century, private mail was stamped with wax. But in the mid to late 20th century, corporate America unwisely switched over to the honor system. Secretive executive messages were simply stuffed into a manila envelope and sealed with a cheap stringy locking mechanism that could be un-spiraled by a dexterous capuchin monkey.

Tim and Dave were just those monkeys.

They, the lowest paid employees at MCF, knew more about what was going on in the agency than many of the six figure earners in their fancy wood-paneled offices.

They knew Jerry in Accounts Receivable was about to be fired for deliberately transposing some numbers and skimming from the top.

They knew the Pizza Shack account was in danger. And that some other agency pitched them some ideas including footage of the most amazing cheese-pulls anyone had ever seen. The Broadcast Department was told, in no uncertain terms, to "get on the horn, pull

out the stops and find us a goddamn shooter who knows how to melt mozzarella!"
And they knew that Wentworth was boning the receptionist, Lucretia, a voluptuous Hispanic girl from El Salvador who could barely speak English.

Tim and Dave both lusted over Lucretia and spent countless hours pondering the exact size and shape of her nipples. Dave confessed that one time his daydreaming about Lucretia got the best of him and he had to slip away downstairs to the loading dock, find a secret corner and unload himself.

"I don't want to open confidential memos, it's depressing."

"Come on. A kid hurled and you had to clean up after it. You think that's never gonna happen again?" said Tim. "This is advertising."

"This is not how I pictured my life after four years of college. Not at all."

You and me both, thought Tim.

"Some day, you'll look back on all this and have a good laugh."

"Some day, huh?"

"Yeah, but for right now I need you to go upstairs to the 8th floor and help Daisy Brown, that junior art director, re-arrange her furniture."

Dave scratched his head.

"I re-arranged her furniture yesterday," he protested.

"She says the light's not good. Wants to re-arrange it again."

Dave shot Tim a look as if to say, "Why don't you do it?"

"I got to make a cigar run. You want to sit on Olympic Blvd. for three hours?"

Before heading up to the 8th floor, Dave grabbed another wedge of juicy orange and started scrubbing his knuckles. The 24 year old had already developed the groan of a man twice his age.

A week later Tim was sorting the updated 11x17 phone lists for the employees of Meehan, Carter and Flears. The lists had to be updated quite regularly as turnover was systemic. They all came and went. Except for the high maintenance prima donnas in the creative department, they never seemed to go anywhere. And why would they, they were treated like kings and queens at MCF.

On the back of the phone lists, the HR department would list the employee monthly birthdays. Accordingly, every other day it seemed like there was some cubicle farm birthday party with a supermarket sheet cake and crappy, fake Martinelli champagne.

Tim never understood why it was the employer's responsibility to throw a sorry soiree on behalf of an associate media planner or a print production coordinator who managed to log another year on planet Earth. Don't these people have friends?

As he curled up the oversized paper so it would fit into the next cubbyhole, he noticed Dave Lang's name on the birthday list.

Tomorrow, his partner in mailroom crime was turning 25. Tim knew this was an opportunity to swing the pendulum, which had recently been dipped in hurled shrimp burrito, in the other direction.

"Happy Birthday, buddddy!" Tim said, as Dave dragged his morning ass into the mailroom.

"Can't wait to see what today has in store. Maybe someone in the research department will have some explosive diarrhea?" Dave shot back.

"Come on, don't be like that. Check it out."

Tim threw him a plastic wrapped copy of *Dairy Cow Monthly*, one of the trade magazines they regularly received because of MCF's representation of Yamaka Tractors, maker of Japan's finest farm equipment. Tim and Dave would spend hours paging through the latest and greatest in bovine news.

It was a way to pass the hours between the mail runs, the furniture schlepping and the million other indignities of being the lowest man on the corporate totem pole.

They'd clip the glossy photos of Jerseys, Holsteins, Pinzgauers, Galloways, Beefmasters, Romagnola and Belgian Blues. And pin them on the mailroom pegboard. Then each would take a turn sexualizing the unknowing beast as if she were a Playmate of the Month.

Clarabelle knows what she wants in a Braford and isn't afraid to say it. She likes long walks in the pasture and the masterful feel of a well-calloused hand on her udders the first thing in the morning.

Dave's mood picked up. Slightly.

"That's just the beginning, my friend. Today you and I are going to Monty's Steakhouse for lunch."

"Come on, you can't afford Monty's."

"You're right, I can't afford Monty's. But Meehan, Carter and Flears can."

Tim unlocked the bottom drawer of his desk, revealing an old tarnished steel lockbox. Inside the lockbox, there was $231.97.

"Holy shit, what is that?"

"Technically it's earmarked for petty cash. Last minute emergencies. Or just some odds and ends for the office. I think rib eye steaks and onion rings are odds and ends, don't you?"

"Isn't someone going to miss the money?"

"They might miss it. If they knew they had it."

"Huh?"

"You know those cigars I buy in K-town for Wentworth?"

"The Cubans?"

"They're not Cubans. They're from Arkansas. Cheap ass ragweed. Made from tobacco even the pigs wouldn't eat. I cozied up to the owner of the cigar store, Kim. He just slaps a fancy Cuban label on them. Then we split the difference."

"You crazy bastard."

"No. That's 'you-crazy-bastard-who's-buying-lunch-today' to you."

Monty's Steakhouse sat atop the Kirby building in Westwood. It had the dark wood and dark leather booths one might expect from a steakhouse. But it also had floor-to-ceiling windows that took full advantage of its southern exposure to the California sun. And, because of its penthouse location, offered panoramic views of the Santa Monica Bay.

On those rare occasions when the UCLA football team beat their crosstown rival, they would celebrate with a carnivorous bacchanalia at Monty's.

The relatively small West Coast financial firms dined there.

And it was frequented by junior agents from CAA and ICM, who had still not learned the ropes, and would pow-wow with their aspiring actresses and writers, who also had still not learned the ropes or made the grade for the tonier restaurants on Melrose or Beverly Hills.

Tim and Dave, in their work shirts and their dungarees, stood out from the crowd sporting Armani and Hugo Boss. But their money – Wentworth's money – was just as good as anybody else's.

"OK, I have two shots of Wild Turkey. And two schooners of pale ale," said Betty, a waitress at Monty's since 1963.

Tim shot back, "Great, can you bring my friend a drink as well?"

"That's good, hun. You boys ready to order?"

She wasn't having any of his schoolboy humor. At this point Tim thought twice about asking for Monty's second most expensive meat stuffed inside their most expensive meat. He and Dave had the #3, rib eye, mashed potatoes and braised mushrooms. They ate like kings and drank like princes.

They downed more Wild Turkey.

Guzzled more beer.

And for dessert, ordered some flambé cake simply because it had rum in it. And because Betty promised to light it on fire.

They packed a night's worth of celebration into a two-hour lunch break. And while some may have called it a day, Tim and Dave were not some. How often, Tim thought, does a man turn 25 years old?

On the short walk back to the office, they passed by the Rathskellar, a chain restaurant fashioned to look and feel like an artisanal microbrewery.

The 34 taps of authentic draft beer proved too tempting. Tim still had a wad of petty cash and by this point in the day's proceedings anything back at the office seemed petty.

Besides, with the exception of Daisy Brown, who wanted her furniture re-arranged again, and perhaps as testament to how little they impacted the agency, nobody missed the boys.

Nobody.

And so they did what two underemployed, over-inebriated, sheepskin-possessing twenty something year olds would do, they drank.

Starting with the stouts and dark beers, they made their way from Ireland across Northern Europe and the various hefeweizens of Bavaria. They tiptoed south through the Baltics and their bitter lagers. From there they traversed the Asian subcontinent, drinking a wide variety of pale ales with their distinctive crisp taste and their notorious high alcohol continent. By the time they had reached Japan they had incurred the wrath of the Rathskellar bartender, who tossed them out and placed them on the Do Not Come Back List.

As they poured out onto the street they passed a gaggle of UCLA sorority sisters from the very snooty Tri-Delt house.

"Hi girls," slurred Dave. They did not even look up at the duo.

"Bye girls," he added.

"Let's go to The Ball," shot Tim.

The Ball was an exclusive gentleman's club. It was invitation only. And because it wasn't open to the public, The Ball was able to skirt California's prudish laws and could serve a full complement of liquor while featuring completely nude dancing girls. Tim and Dave wisely did not get in their cars and instead began the mile and a half walk towards Santa Monica.

Redemption in Guanajuato, Mexico

A long walk for a short drink.

A 300 pound man wearing a blazer that was three sizes too small for his massive chest stood between the boys and the magic combination of full nudity and a full bar.

"Members only," he barked.

"That's alright, I'm friends with Frank. He told us to meet him here," Tim adlibbed.

"Frank? Unless your friend Frank is standing right here with a membership card in his hand, you're not going in there," he pointed to the oasis beyond the curtain.

Tim tried to stick his head in to look for his imaginary friend Frank. And to sneak a peak at some unsheathed boobs.

"Touch that velvet curtain again and they'll be wrapping you in it at your funeral."

"Is that so?" asked Tim, who mistakenly believed he could outwit this lunkhead.

The bouncer looked over the two skinny mailroom clerks and pronounced, "Oh that is most assuredly *so*."

His command of a four-syllable word, plus the size of his fists, roughly a large canned ham, were quite convincing.

Drunk, horny, and angry, now angrier, the two mailroom clerks made the long walk back to Westwood.

They began talking shop. That is, they resumed talking shop. For a short while they were talking about tits and asses, but that didn't come to fruition, so they went to the default conversation about Meehan, Carter and Flears.

And they couldn't talk MCF without mentioning Wentworth.

"I'll bet Wentworth has a membership at The Ball."

"I hate that bastard."

"I'm past hating him. I hate broccoli and cats. I detest Wentworth. I loathe him. There are days I can't even speak his name. He's not fit to breath the same air as the rest of us. If his body was on fire I'd break out the chocolate, marshmallows and graham crackers."

As they made their way past the unkempt grounds of the Veteran Center on Wilshire Blvd., Dave spotted something.

"I have an idea." Dave turned to Tim, "You have the keys to the office?"

Tim pulled up his loose shirttail, revealing an odd assortment of 27 keys attached to his belt loop.

Dave, looked around, spotted a nearby garbage can, reached in and pulled out a small plastic bag.

"What have you got in mind?" asked Tim.

"Something monumental!" said Dave.

On Monday morning, the office was buzzing. Gasps and groans could be heard around every corner.

"Oh my god!"

"I can't believe it!"

"Are you sure?"

"No way."

"Way!"

In the coffee room, many of the secretaries gathered around Elizabeth Robbins, who was Bill Wentworth's executive secretary. She rarely had the opportunity to hold court, but today's activities put her front and center, and she relished the attention.

She poured herself a second cup of coffee and delivered a graphic blow-by-blow account.

"Mr. Wentworth was searching for his favorite letter opener. He has three. But he likes to use the one given to him by President Reagan at that golf tournament fundraiser. So I tell him to look in the upper drawer of his credenza, which is locked. So now he has to find the key. And I don't have it. Only the mailroom guys and the janitorial staff have the key. He starts looking around. Can't find the key. Starts getting all huffy and puffy. I tell him to check the pocket on the extra blazer he keeps on the hook of his door in case there's an emergency meeting."

"Found it," he yells.

"So Mr. Wentworth opens the top drawer of the credenza, hoping to find his special Ronald Reagan Presidential Letter Opener, but what does he find instead?"

By now, the other secretaries have leaned in and are hanging on her every word.

"He finds dog shit. Five pounds of perfectly coiled, still somewhat fresh, dog shit."

"Get out!"

Redemption in Guanajuato, Mexico

"Looked like it came from the ass of a Great Dane. Or a St. Bernard. Or a one of those big Bernese Mountain Hound Dogs. It was huge. And smelly. Did I mention it was huge? I swear if I didn't know better it could have come from a man."

"What did Mr. Wentworth do?"

"I've seen him mad before. But this was different. This was like a quiet, scary mad. He bit his lips, walked down the hallway straight down to Mr. Meehan's office. All I heard was a door slam."

There was going to be hell to pay.

And Tim and Dave were sure they would be picking up the tab.

Their once not-so-promising start in advertising had become even less promising. Tim pictured himself back at his old job, assembling wheelchairs and crutches at a factory in West Covina.

Dave could return to the local restaurants, where there was always a need for a fast moving line cook. Their career vectors would have to be recalculated. All because of a drunken bender and the unwise decision to render unto Caesar that which belonged to Caesar.

But the axe fell elsewhere.

Flacco Fernandez, the proud janitor who had previous run-ins with Bill Wentworth, was fingered as the culprit. And though there was no evidence, it was clear he had the motive. He had the opportunity. And he had the key to Wentworth's desk drawer.

He was told to clean out his locker and find a menial underpaying job elsewhere. He never did. In fact, Flacco was never heard from or seen by anyone in Los Angeles ever again.

Redemption in Guanajuato, Mexico

Tim and Dave spent another year in that mailroom. They groused and grumbled but finally got off their asses. And with the help of some of the creatives at MCF, put a portfolio together.

Tim got out first, landing a job writing ads for a local Fruit of the Month delivery service. Dave exited shortly thereafter, penning ads for a maker of premium fishing gear, salt and freshwater.

It wasn't ideal for either, but it wasn't hauling boxes and it wasn't running interference for one of the legendary assholes in the Southern California ad community.

They had their start. And they made the most of it. Parlaying a career in advertising to a few stints in television. For three years they were show runners on *There's a Monkey on My Back*. When that ran its course, they put their minds together and wrote several movie scripts including a film that went on to become a yearly action-adventure franchise.

It all generated residuals. Years of mailbox money. Residuals that may never have been, had they paid the cost for one fateful Friday night.

Guanajuato is a small village in central Mexico.

It is inhabited by 937 people, including Flacco Fernandez, the former janitor who returned here more than 30 years ago.

Flacco married his teenage *novia*, Maria, and together they have six children. As a guitarist in a mariachi band he doesn't make great money, just enough to put a roof over his family's head and put food on the table.

To some it may not be much; but to Flacco it is more than enough.

On a rainy, sticky afternoon, a monsoonal tropical storm blows through Guanajuato. Nothing serious, just enough to dislodge some

184

palm fronds from the trees and tip over a wheelbarrow or two. Flacco steps out of his modest adobe home to retrieve the mail.

There, he finds a small package from *Los Estados Unidos*. There was not much of a return address; it simply said it was from Warner Brothers Studios in Burbank, California. Inside the package, there were two items. One was an envelope, containing a money order made out to Flacco. A money order for $10,000.

Flacco could not believe it. His eyes danced around. Was this part of some sting? Was somebody setting him up? What is the meaning of all this?

He decided to wait a week. Caution, he thought, was his best approach. He waited another week, nothing happened.

Then he quietly deposited the money order for $10,000, an enormous sum of money that could sustain him and his family for the rest of his years in Guanajuato.

He withdrew $50 and found himself a seat at Estevan's, an open-air bar under a giant palapa set amongst the beautiful rainforest trees in Central Mexico.

He ordered himself a pint of Estevan's coldest *cerveza*. And a double shot of Siembra Azul artisanal tequila made from 100% blue agave.

And then he indulged himself with the other contents of the mystery package from Los Angeles. He popped the cap off a small mailing tube. Undid the wrapper. And savored the freshly released aroma.

Then, Flacco lit up an authentic Domingo Robusto, a thick torpedo shaped cigar from Havana, Cuba.

EPILOGUE

I can't recall the epilogue of any book I've ever read. I dare say, you'd have a hard time as well. I suspect that after turning the last page of a story, or a collection of highly fictionalized stories devoid of any defamation or slander, most people shut the covers, and move on.

After all, there are Kardashians to be kept up with, tweets to be re-tweeted and data-rich browser histories to be erased.

Of course, as you can see, that's not going to stop me from writing an epilogue. Just as common sense, a pile of literary agent rejection letters and the very real possibility that I will never work in the advertising industry again didn't stop me from writing this book.

Which begs the question, at least from my wife, why sink good hard-earned money into a book of sophomoric stories no one outside of advertising will read? It's like tossing cash in the toilet.

Only it isn't.

You see, I know advertising people. I know their strengths, their weaknesses and their boundless egos. Boundless.

I also know people in advertising make it a habit to Google their names at least two to three times a week.

Knowing all this, and based solely on the inherent narcissism of friends and colleagues in the industry, I can safely predict the release of this micro-niche book about advertising and the people who create it, is good for a thousand, maybe two thousand, immediate sales.

Easy.

They'll want to know if I've written about them. Or, even as the title indicates with the names changed and such, they'll want to see if they can recognize any of the situations or characters laid out in the dozen stories.

And that is just a small subset of a larger potential market.

Winston Churchill famously said, "You have enemies? Good. That means you stood up for something, sometime in your life."

As you might have guessed, the number of people I call friends and colleagues in the business is far outnumbered by the people who might consider me an enemy.

Over the course of my 25 years in the industry, with long term as well as short-term gigs at almost every ad agency that ever hung a shingle, I've made it a practice to stand up for something.

It might have been a headline. An idea. A platform. A concept. A campaign. But chances are, if I felt strongly about it, I went to bat for it.

I could have, and probably should have, been more diplomatic and as a result, been way more effective. But that's the type of wisdom that is forged with hindsight, two pressing mortgages and a nagging feeling of professional underachievement.

I can't do anything about it now, nor do I want to. I'm tired.

But I can tally up the number of planners, account executives, former partners, ex-bosses, clients and put-out-to-pasture CEO's, with whom I have tangled in the past, and know if they have any inkling that I've written about them, they're going to be the first ones logging onto amazon.com with their credit card in hand. And Priority shipping on their mind.

That's the power of Ego.

If I've done the math right, I could make a few bucks with this book.

If I haven't done the math right, and there's a better chance of that, I'll be in the hole for a bit. Nothing I can't skim off the top of my daughter's 529 college savings account.

Either way, I hope you had half as much fun reading it, as I had writing it.

See you over at roundseventeen.blogspot.com.

ABOUT THE AUTHOR

Rich Siegel is a freelance copywriter, blogger, former group creative director, part time screenwriter and a full time father of two daughters.

His previous book *Tuesdays With Mantu, My Adventures with a Nigerian Con Artist* (tuesdayswithmantu.com) won no awards, earned little in the way of literary recognition, but has been surprisingly incorporated into several college curriculums regarding Internet scamming.

Rich and his art director partner, John Shirley, are best recognized for ABC's breakthrough *Yellow* Campaign which turned the network broadcasting industry on its head from 1997 to 1999. And earned an estimated $12 million worth of free publicity, $3 million of it was good.

They also created and co-executive produced Home Movie, a full-length documentary about five eccentric families and how they have redefined the American dream of home ownership.

Rich spent the majority of his advertising career at Chiat/Day and has put in considerable time at many of the world's largest agencies, including: BBDO, DDB, Saatchi & Saatchi, Y&R, JWT, McCann Erikson, Deutsch, and many more.

When not swimming, biking or hiking, and not fighting with his bi-polar neighbor about his cantankerous dog, Rich likes to poke fun at Kim Jung Un, Dear Leader of the People's Republic of North Korea (Korea's best Korea) at http://kimjungfun.tumblr.com.

APPRECIATION

Special thanks go out to Robert Prins for his amazing cover design. To Henry Hsu for his design and photo assistance. To Rachel Plecas for proofreading. To Bob Hoffman, the *Ad Contrarian*, for his help, and for putting me in touch with Bonnie Miguel, a formatting force to be reckoned with.

And thanks to friends, family, fellow bloggers and colleagues who encouraged me to stop playing online chess and do something useful.

And extra special thanks to my wife Debbie, who is and will always be, a saint. My saint.

Now, I will take out the garbage.

www.ingramcontent.com/pod-product-compliance
Lightning Source LLC
Chambersburg PA
CBHW060847280326
41934CB00007B/949